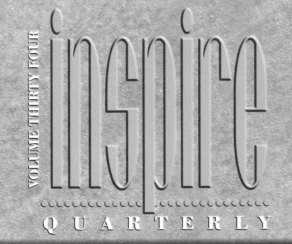

VOLUME THIRTY FOUR

inspire

QUARTERLY

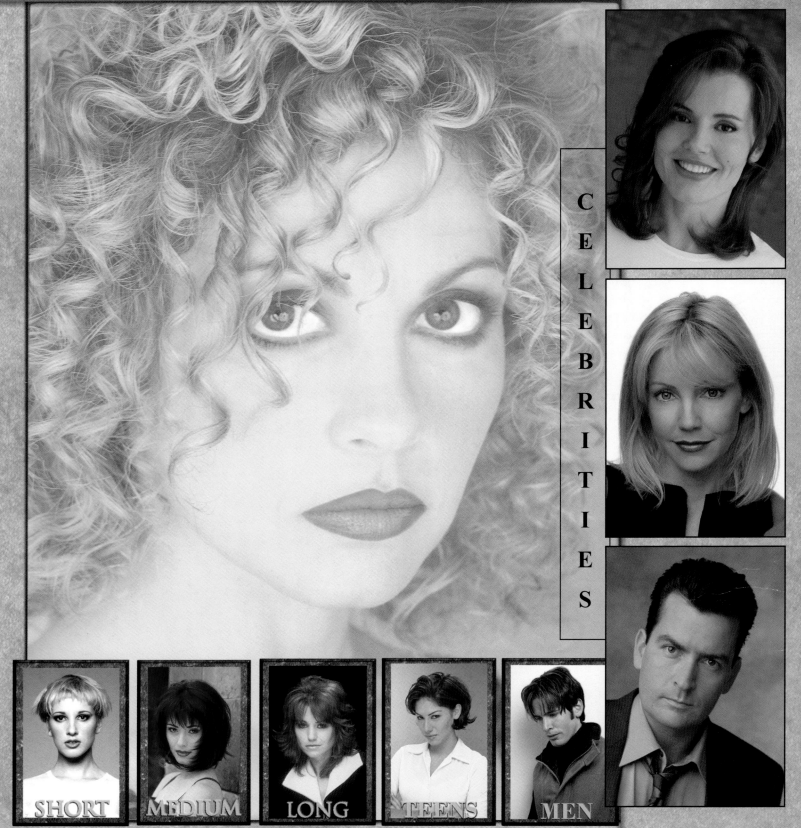

C E L E B R I T I E S

SHORT MEDIUM LONG TEENS MEN

Graphic Design by Androniki Saravis

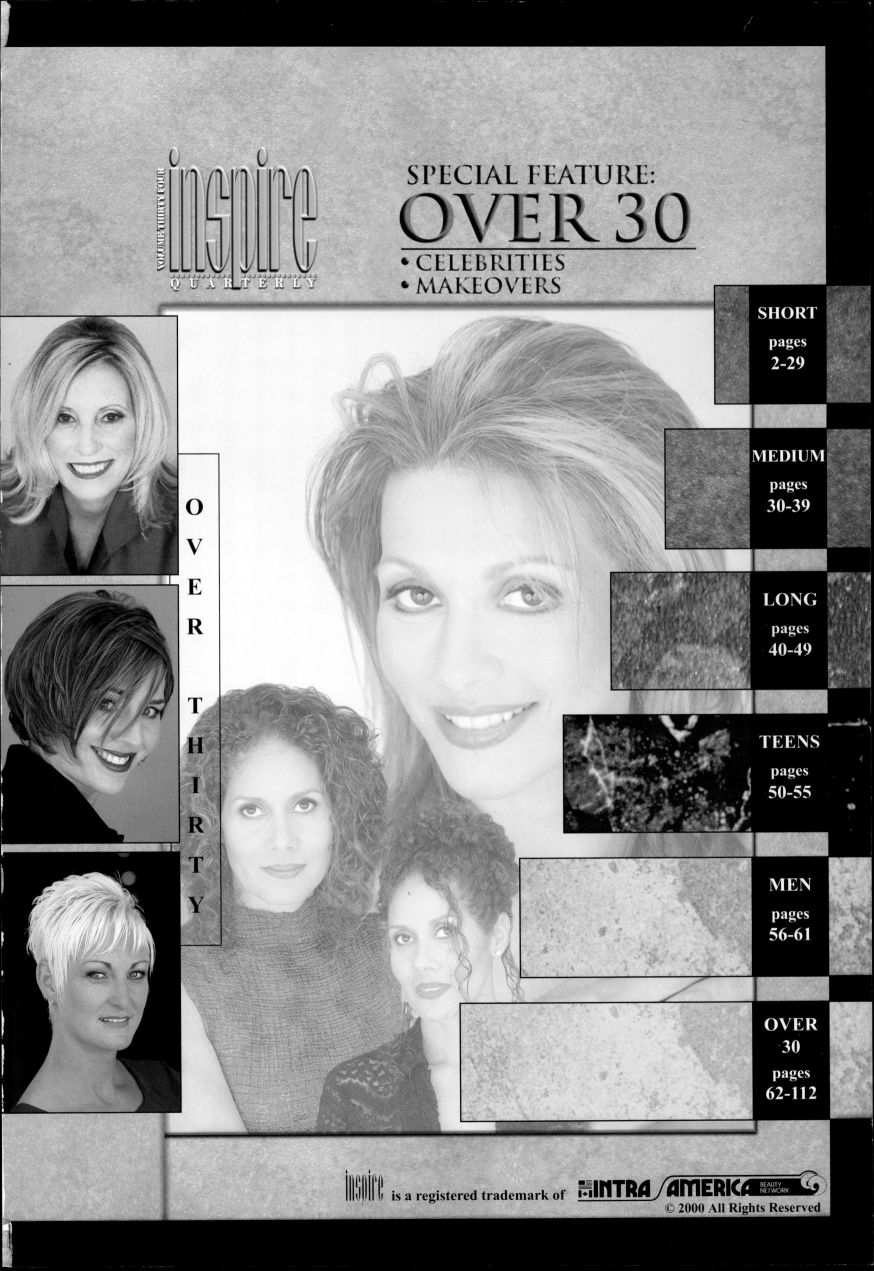

VOLUME THIRTY FOUR

inspire
QUARTERLY

SPECIAL FEATURE:
OVER 30
- CELEBRITIES
- MAKEOVERS

OVER THIRTY

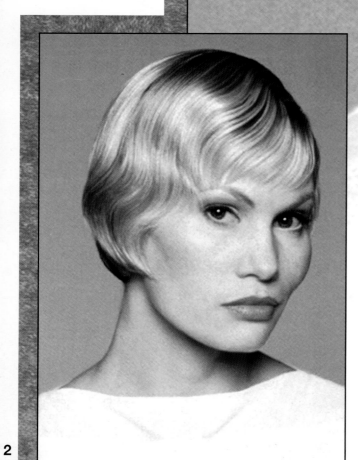

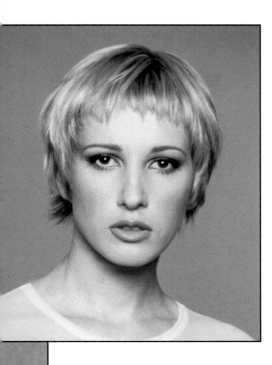

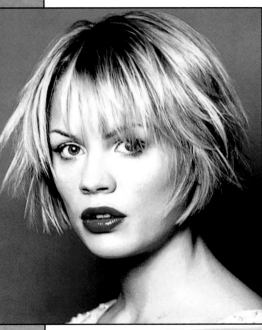

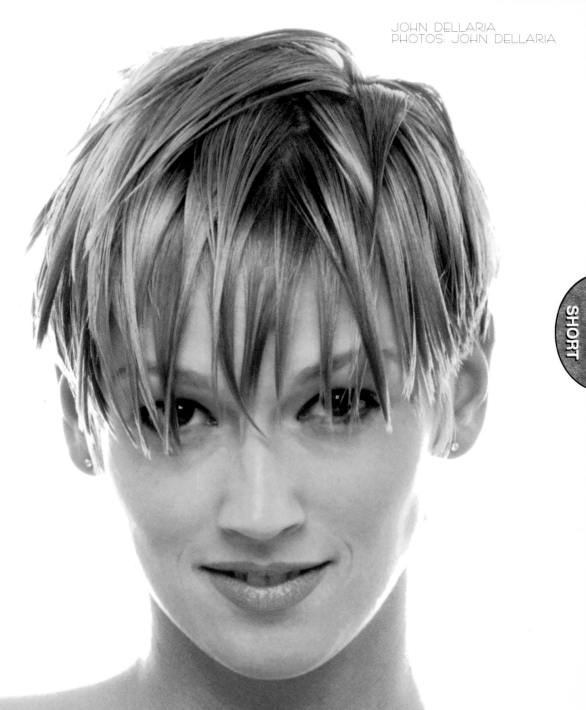

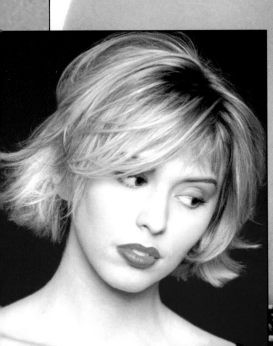

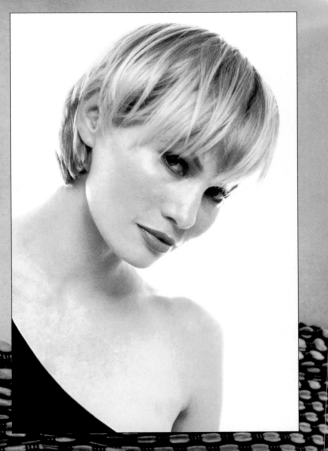

Is there water on the moon?

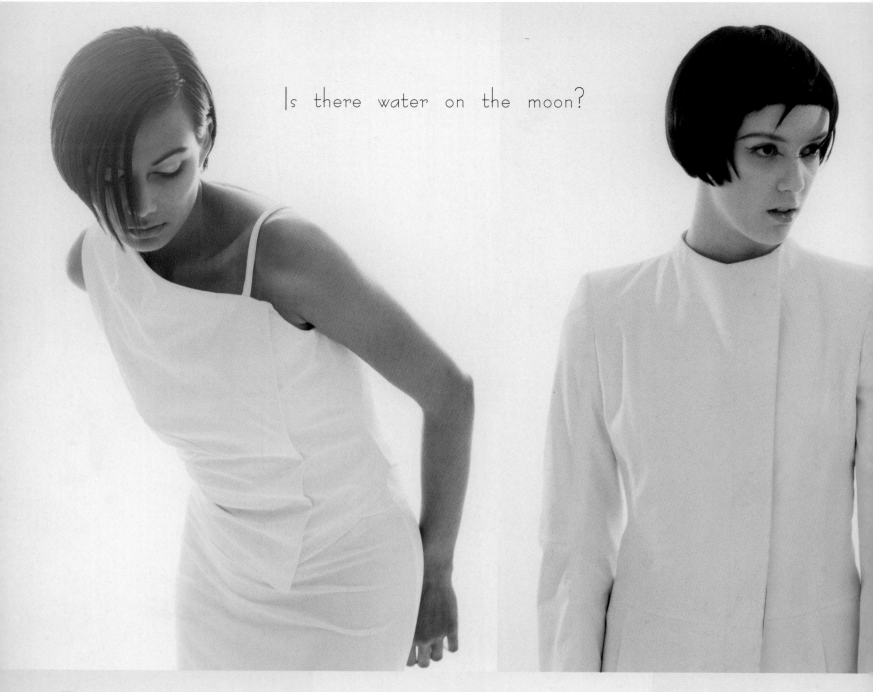

The collection was inspired by the serenity and tranquillity of space, and the evolvement of raw feminini

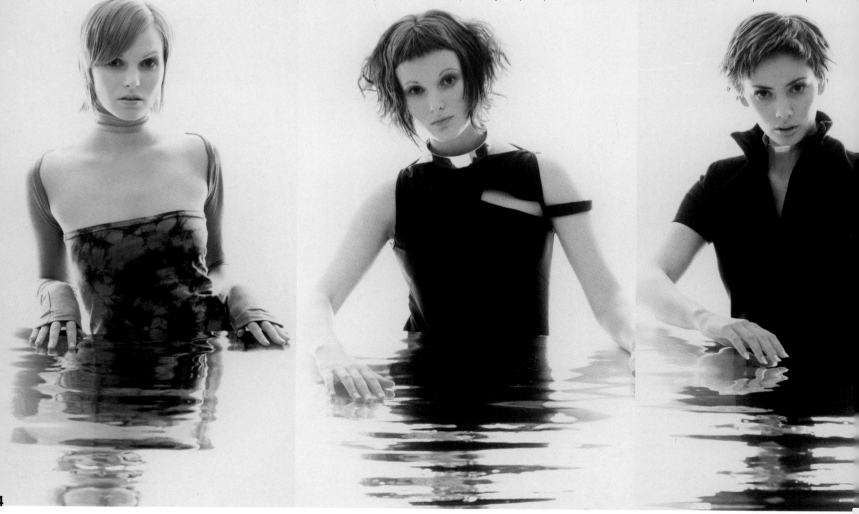

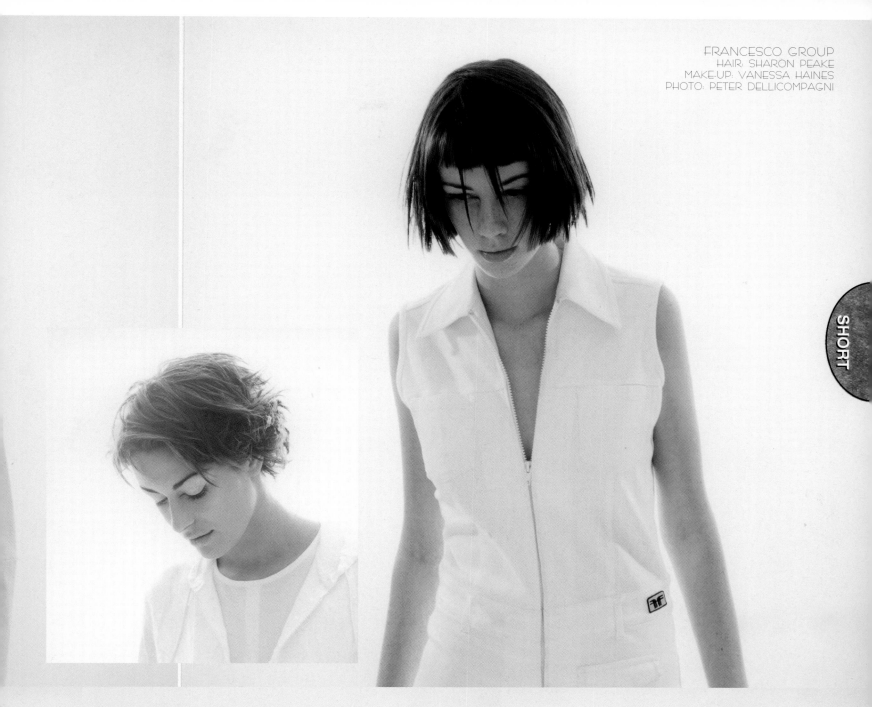

FRANCESCO GROUP
HAIR: SHARON PEAKE
MAKE-UP: VANESSA HAINES
PHOTO: PETER DELLICOMPAGNI

SHORT

fresh individualism for a new era.   - Francesco Group

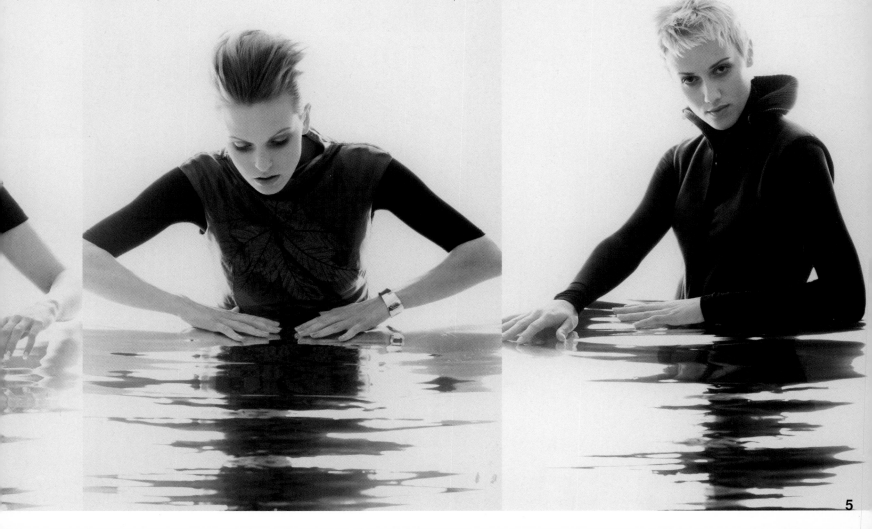

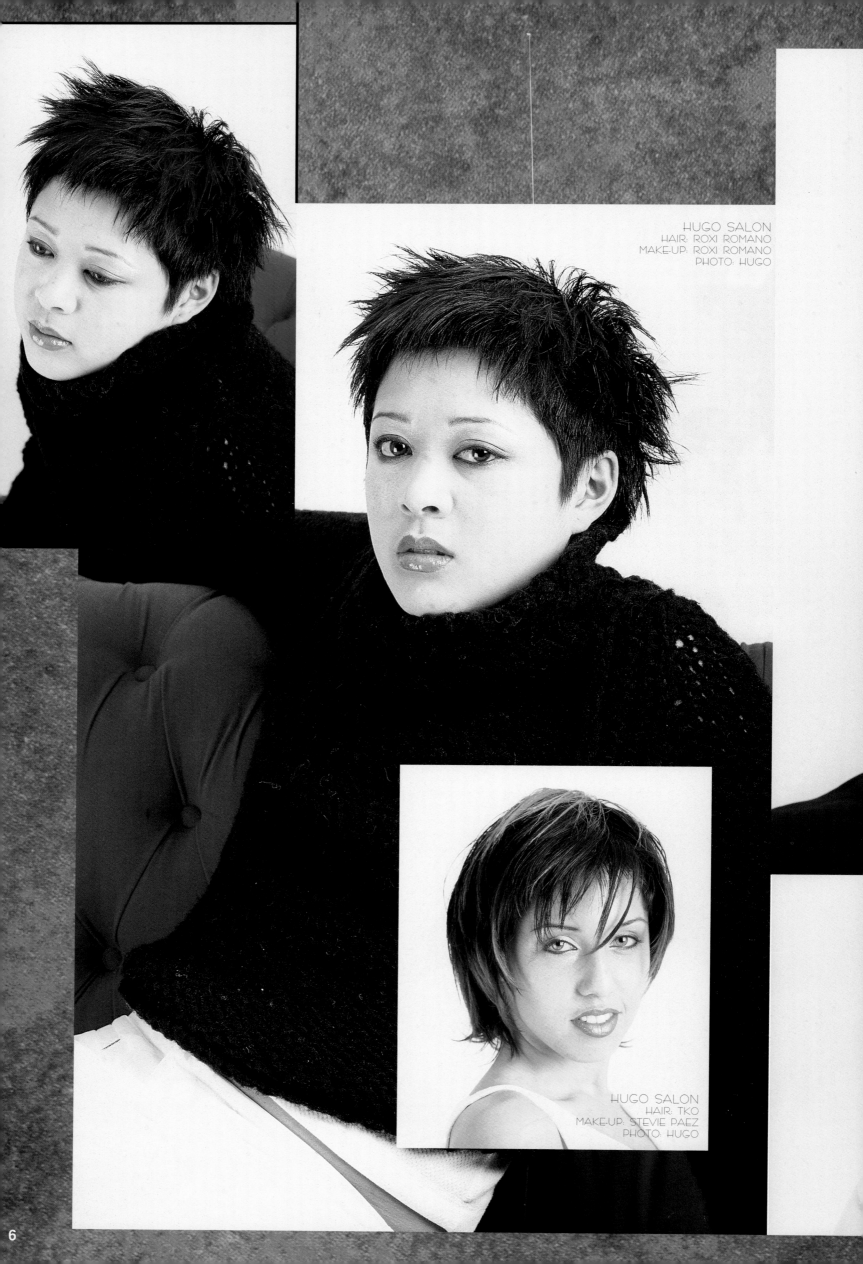

HUGO SALON
HAIR: ROXI ROMANO
MAKE-UP: ROXI ROMANO
PHOTO: HUGO

HUGO SALON
HAIR: TKO
MAKE-UP: STEVIE PAEZ
PHOTO: HUGO

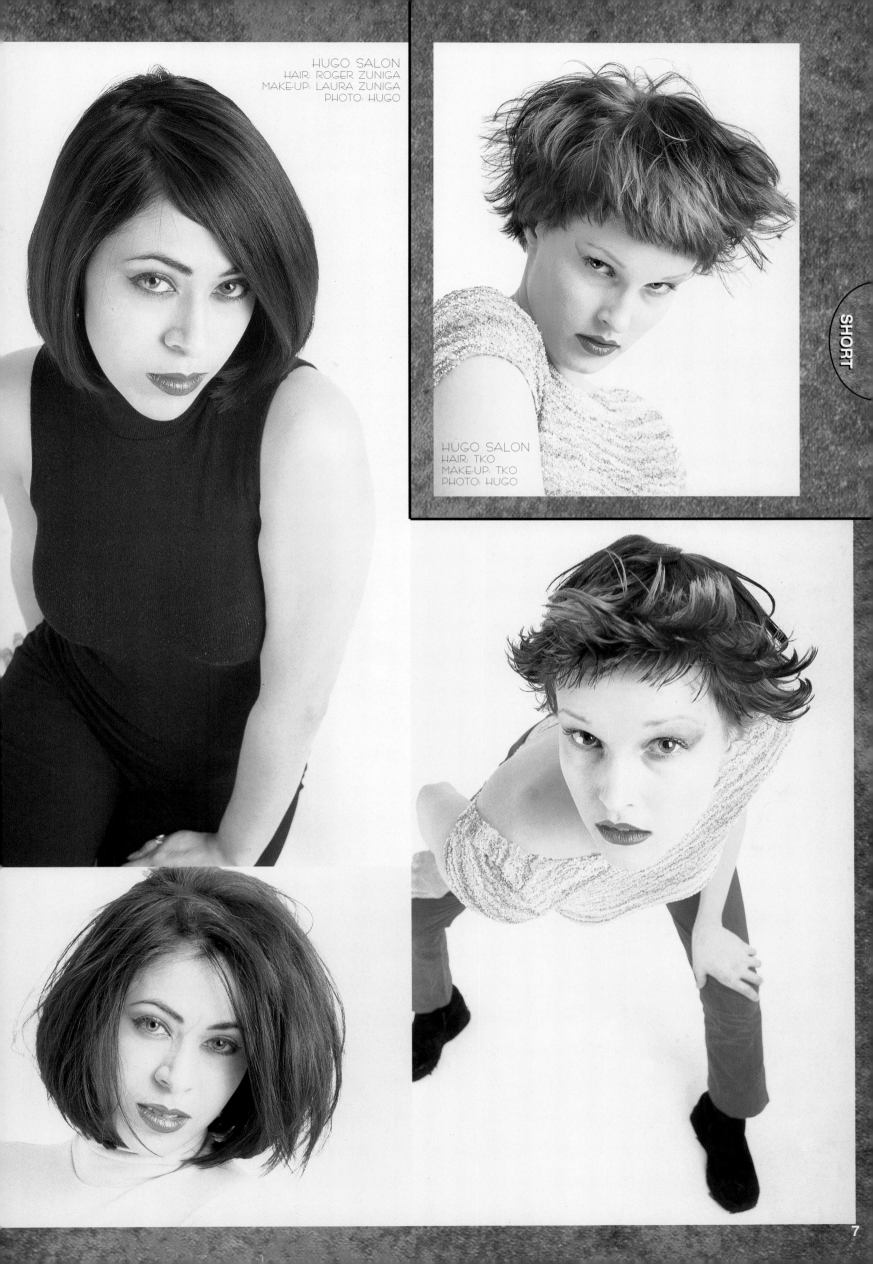

HUGO SALON
HAIR: ROGER ZUNIGA
MAKE-UP: LAURA ZUNIGA
PHOTO: HUGO

HUGO SALON
HAIR: TKO
MAKE-UP: TKO
PHOTO: HUGO

ROCCO ALTOBELLI
HAIR: NINO ALTOBELLI & WILLIAM ANDERSON

Rocco Altobelli Salons
& Day Spas
have created a new spin on a classic, dependable style.

Altobelli's New Generation Bob is a thoroughly modern version of the bi-level bob... textured, feminine and definitely flirty...

it's in charge for Fall of 2000, it's kicky, fringy and funky.

ROCCO ALTOBELLI
HAIR: NINO ALTOBELLI & WILLIAM ANDERSON

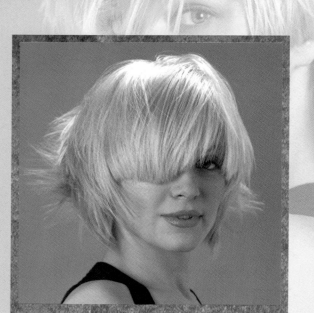

ROCCO ALTOBELLI
HAIR: JULIE GJOVIK & WILLIAM ANDERSON

ROCCO ALTOBELLI
HAIR: JULIE GJOVIK & WILLIAM ANDERSON

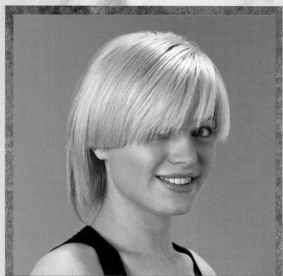

ROCCO ALTOBELLI
HAIR: JULIE GJOVIK & WILLIAM ANDERSON

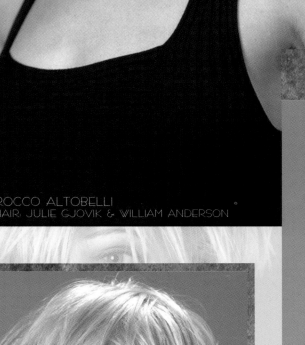

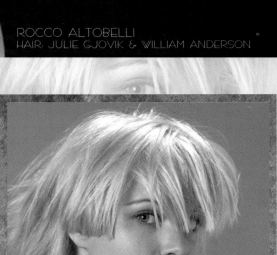

ROCCO ALTOBELLI
HAIR: JULIE GJOVIK & WILLIAM ANDERSON

ROCCO ALTOBELLI
HAIR: JULIE GJOVIK & WILLIAM ANDERSON

9

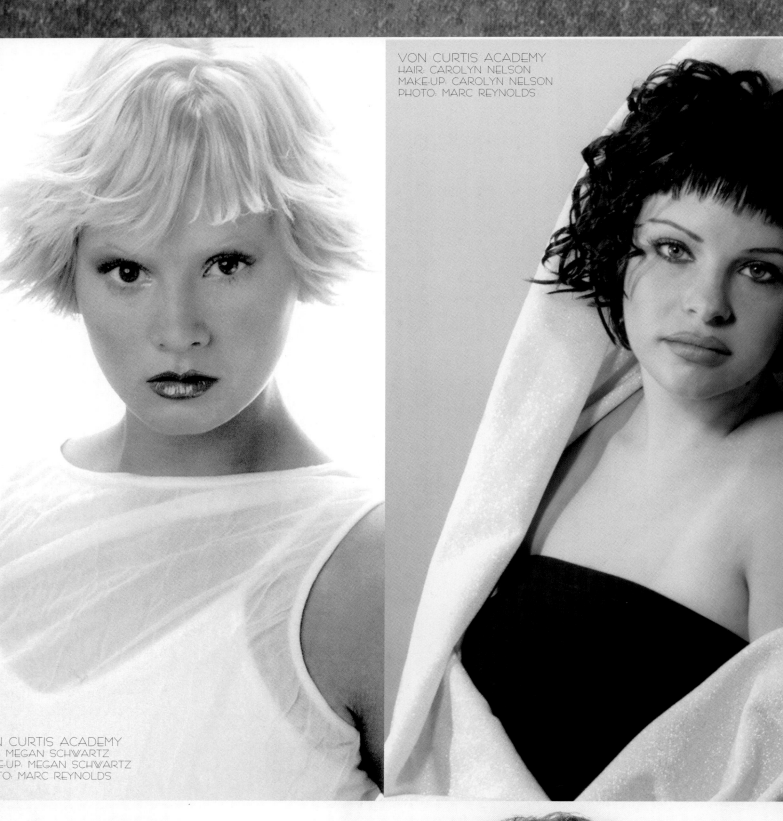

VON CURTIS ACADEMY
HAIR: CAROLYN NELSON
MAKE-UP: CAROLYN NELSON
PHOTO: MARC REYNOLDS

VON CURTIS ACADEMY
HAIR: MEGAN SCHWARTZ
MAKE-UP: MEGAN SCHWARTZ
PHOTO: MARC REYNOLDS

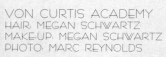

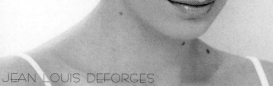

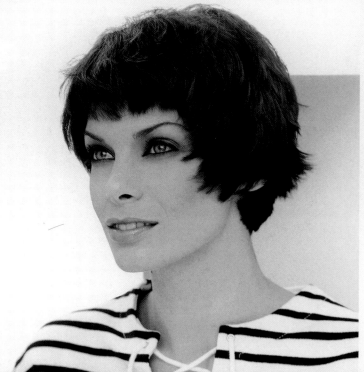

JEAN LOUIS DEFORGES

The concept is casual and natural,
softer, younger, sexier.
Hair is uniquely personalized
to the individual.

-DeBerardinis

VON CURTIS ACADMY
HAIR: CAROLYN NELSON
MAKE-UP: CAROLYN NELSON
PHOTO: MARC REYNOLDS

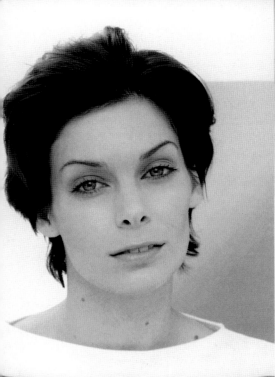

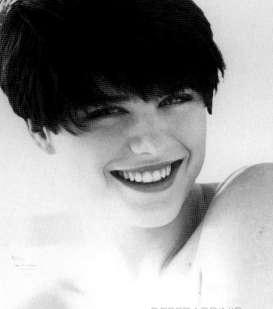

DEBERARDINIS

DEBERARDINIS

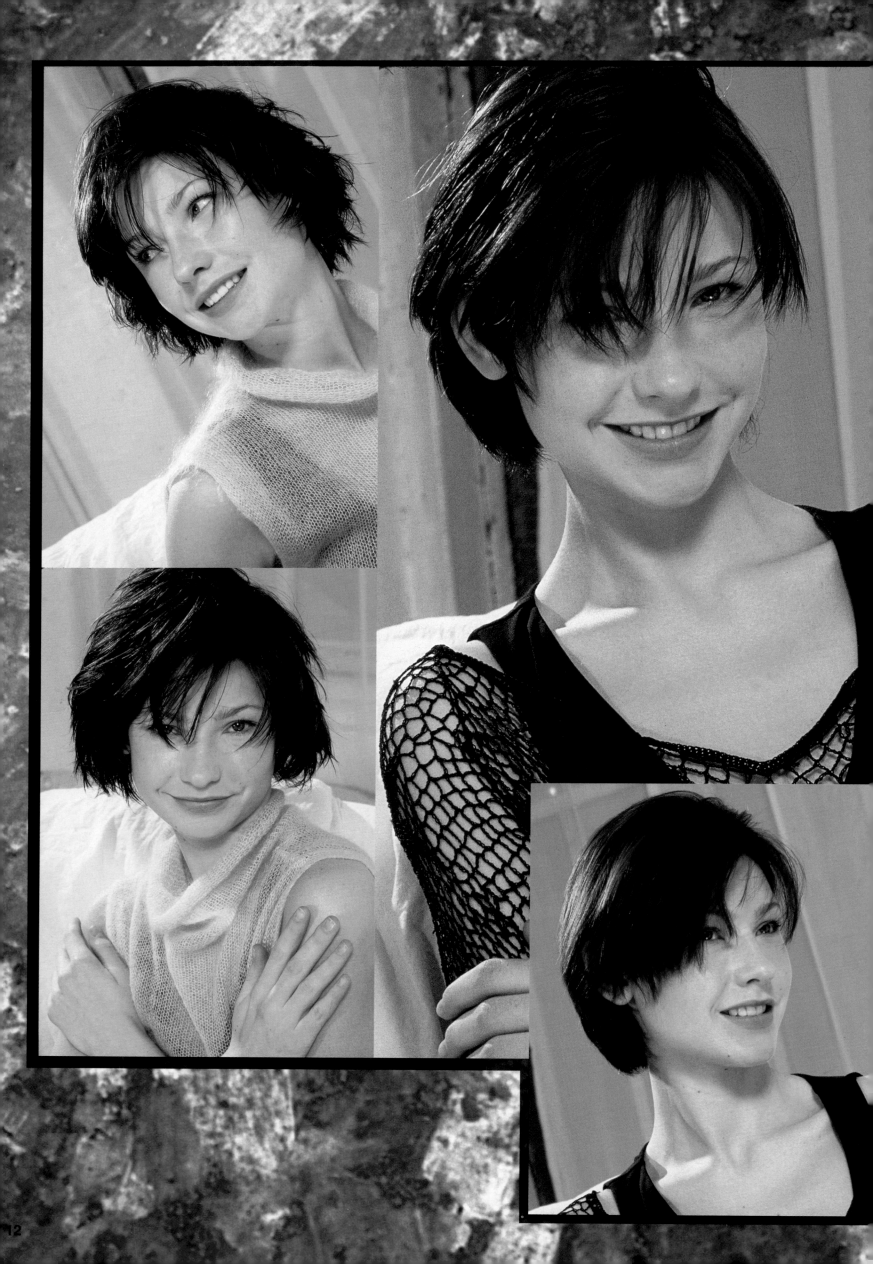

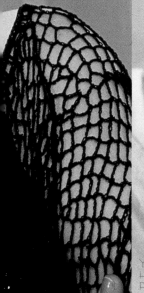

For this collection my emphasis was on creating soft edges at the ends of the hairstyles. I designed an untamed messy look to display the active motion and the exciting flow of hair.
Yosh Toya

YOSH FOR HAIR
HAIR: YOSH TOYA
PHOTO: BARRY YEE

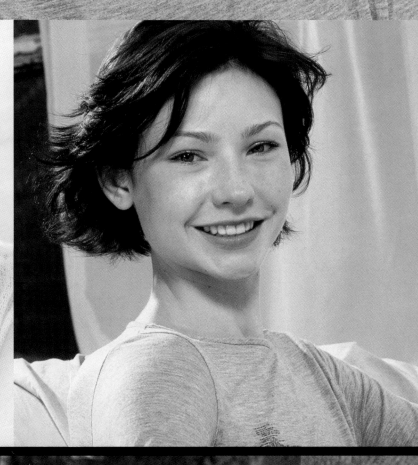

YOSH FOR HAIR
HAIR: YOSH TOYA
MAKE-UP: OLESYA
PHOTO: BARRY YEE

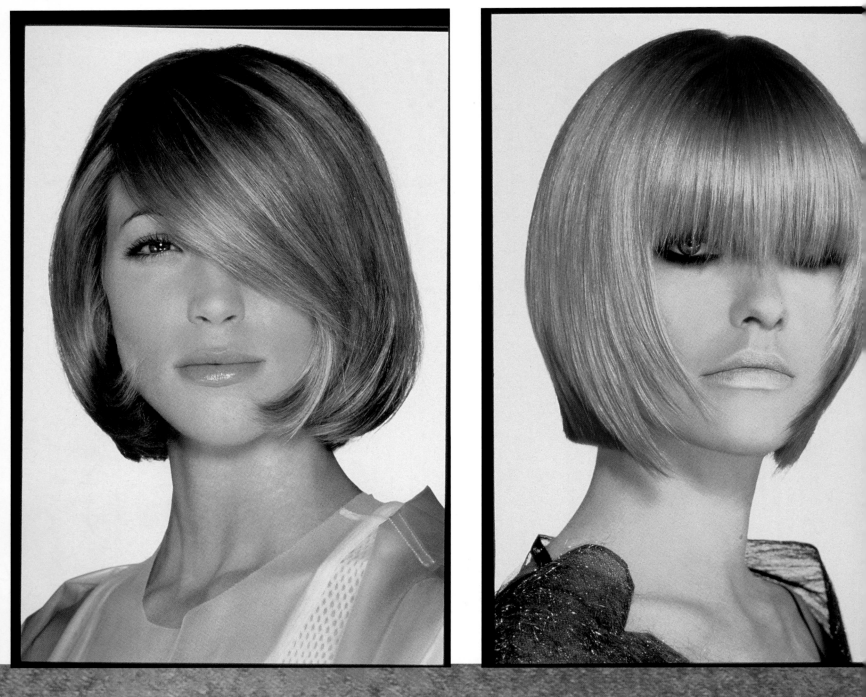

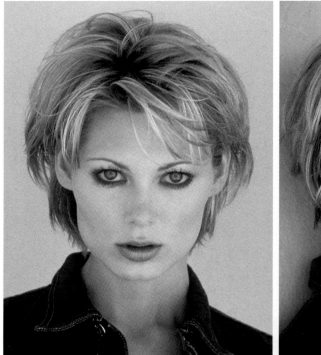

DON SHAW HAIRDRESSERS
HAIR: DIMITRIOS NICOLAOU
MAKE-UP: SYLVIA SHAW
PHOTO: AKIN GIRAV

What's New, What's Hot, What's Hairstyle?

Function, Fun, Flirting and Folly.

FUNCTION – basic, clean, easy-to-manage

FAMILY – traditional, cozy, romantic

FLIRTING – seductive, elegant, festive

FOLLY – crazy, floral, creative

Don Shaw Hairdressers

This look was created by drying the hair and then cutting by taking sections of the hair with a seven-row natural bristle brush instead of a comb. Picking up the section of dry hair with a bristle brush breaks it up a bit and it still remains versatile. A gel and oil was mixed together to position the hair.

Dimitrios Nicolaou

DON SHAW HAIRDRESSERS
HAIR: DIMITRIOS NICOLAOU
MAKE-UP: SYLVIA SHAW
PHOTO: AKIN GIRAV

15

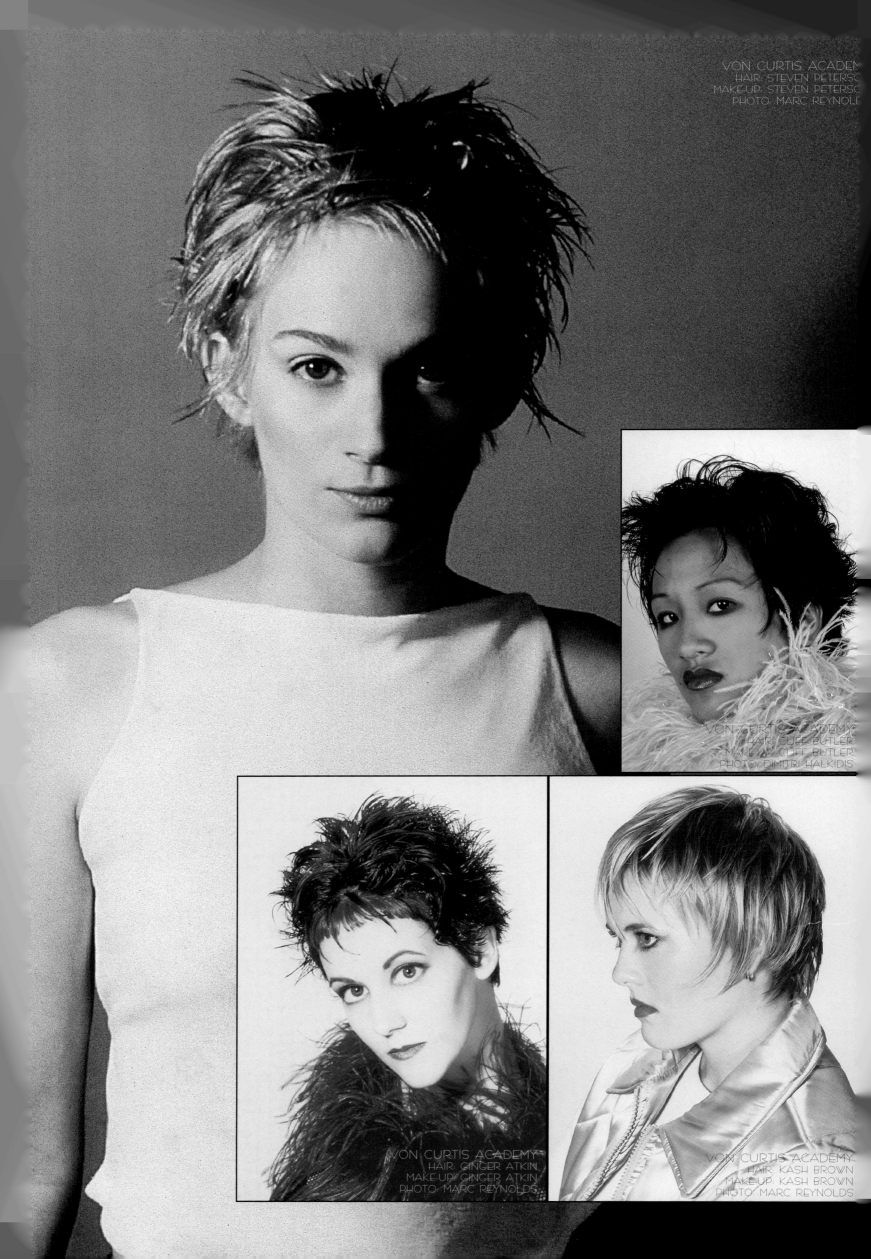

VON CURTIS ACADEMY
HAIR: STEVEN PETERSON
MAKE-UP: STEVEN PETERSON
PHOTO: MARC REYNOLDS

VON CURTIS ACADEMY
HAIR: KASH BROWN
MAKE-UP: KASH BROWN
PHOTO: MARC REYNOLDS

VON CURTIS ACADEMY
HAIR: CLIFF BUTLER
MAKE-UP: CLIFF BUTLER
PHOTO: DIMITRI HALKIDIS

VON CURTIS ACADEMY
HAIR: GINGER ATKIN
MAKE-UP: GINGER ATKIN
PHOTO: MARC REYNOLDS

VON CURTIS ACADEMY
HAIR: KASH BROWN
MAKE-UP: KASH BROWN
PHOTO: MARC REYNOLDS

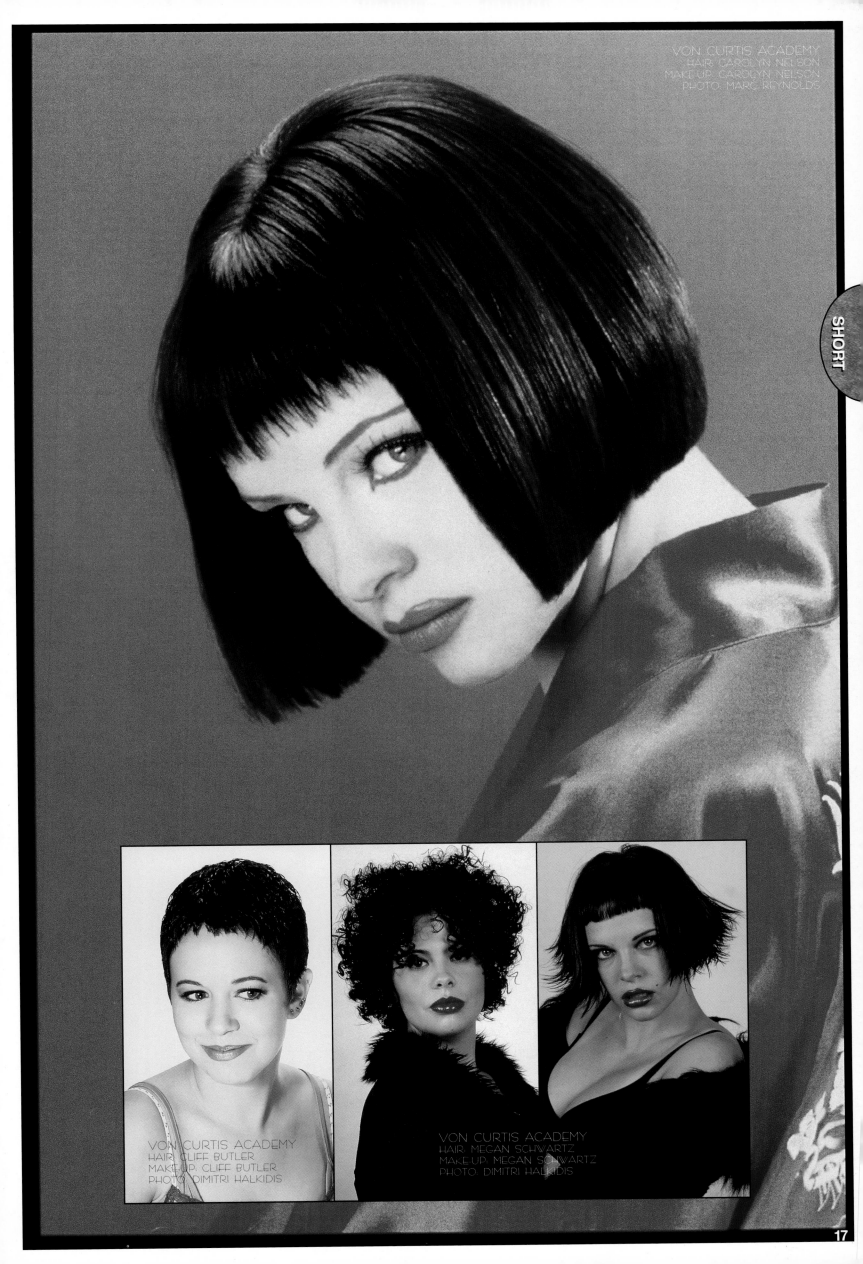

VON CURTIS ACADEMY
HAIR: CAROLYN NELSON
MAKE-UP: CAROLYN NELSON
PHOTO: MARC REYNOLDS

VON CURTIS ACADEMY
HAIR: CLIFF BUTLER
MAKE-UP: CLIFF BUTLER
PHOTO: DIMITRI HALKIDIS

VON CURTIS ACADEMY
HAIR: MEGAN SCHWARTZ
MAKE-UP: MEGAN SCHWARTZ
PHOTO: DIMITRI HALKIDIS

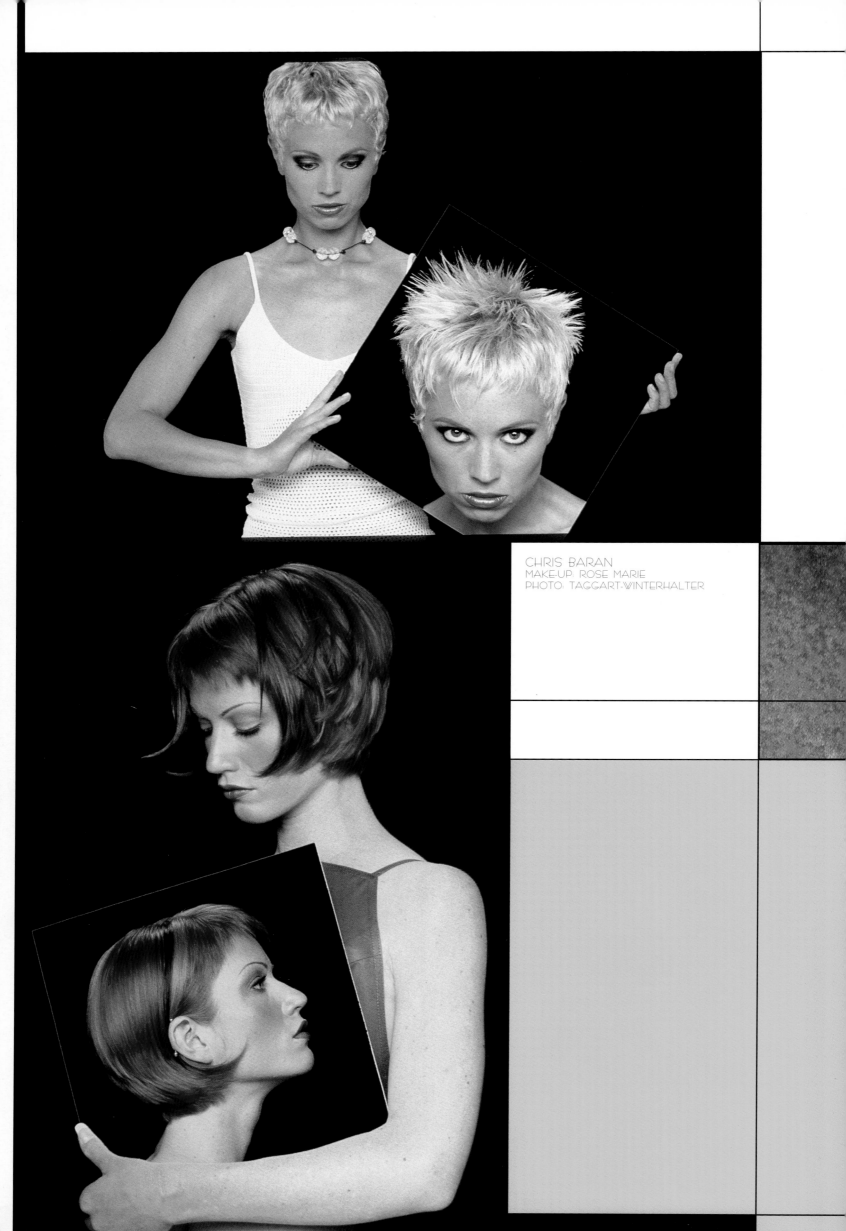

CHRIS BARAN
MAKE-UP: ROSE MARIE
PHOTO: TAGGART-WINTERHALTER

Studio Ricera Moda

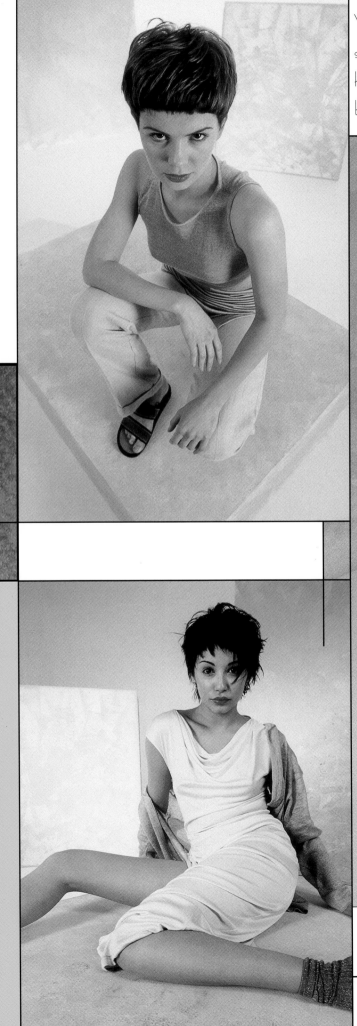

Who needs boring brown? Dark Blond Tobacco looks soft and natural, and gets a touch of vibrancy from blond highlights that hold their tone against the sun better because they're permanent.

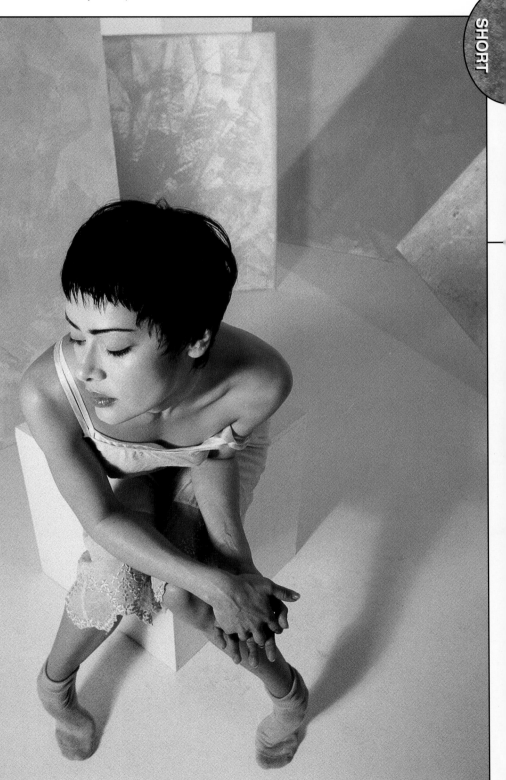

STUDIO RICERA MODA
HAIR: STUDIO RICERA MODA
MAKE-UP: STUDIO RICERA MODA
PHOTO: LEONARDO BAGAGLI

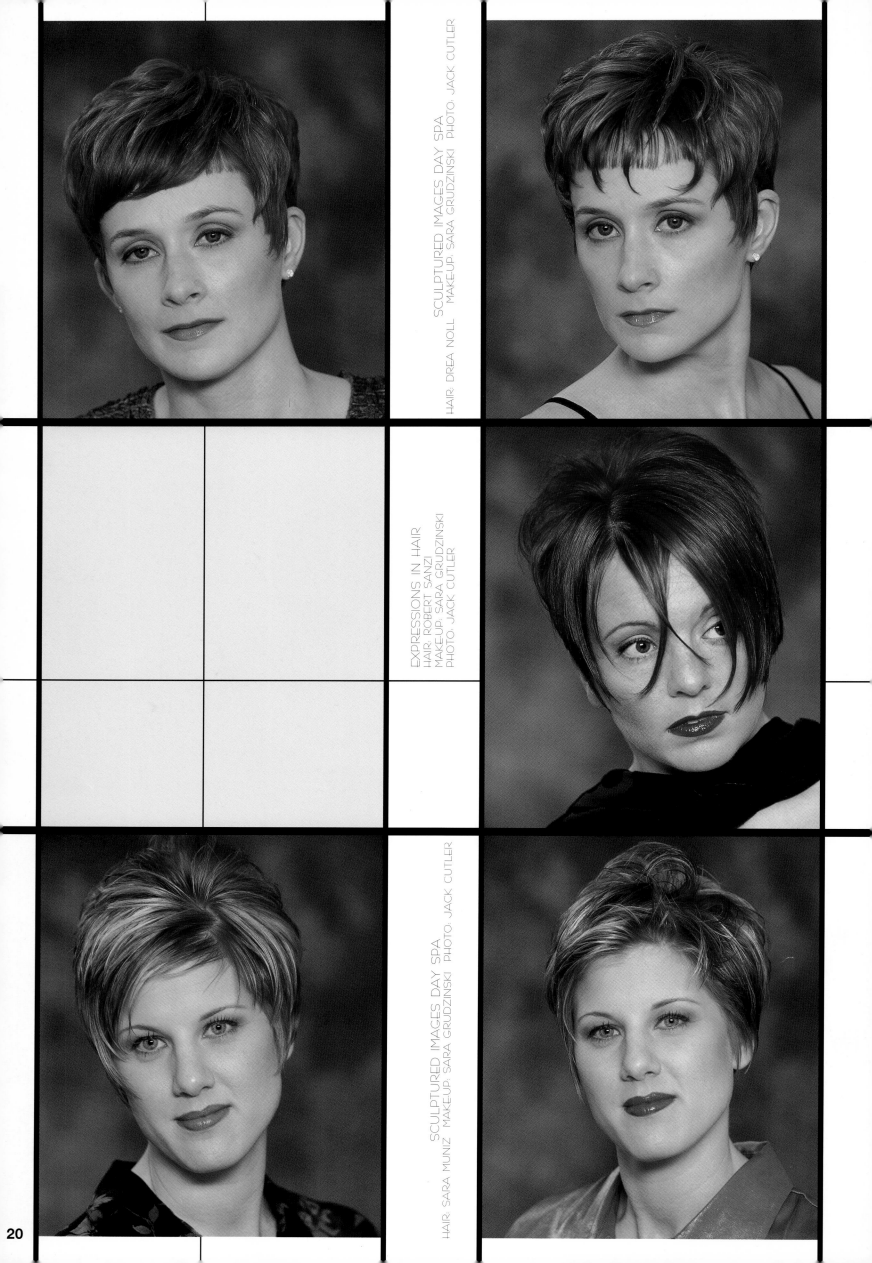

SCULPTURED IMAGES DAY SPA
HAIR: DREA NOLL   MAKEUP: SARA GRUDZINSKI   PHOTO: JACK CUTLER

EXPRESSIONS IN HAIR
HAIR: ROBERT SANZI
MAKEUP: SARA GRUDZINSKI
PHOTO: JACK CUTLER

SCULPTURED IMAGES DAY SPA
HAIR: SARA MUNIZ   MAKEUP: SARA GRUDZINSKI   PHOTO: JACK CUTLER

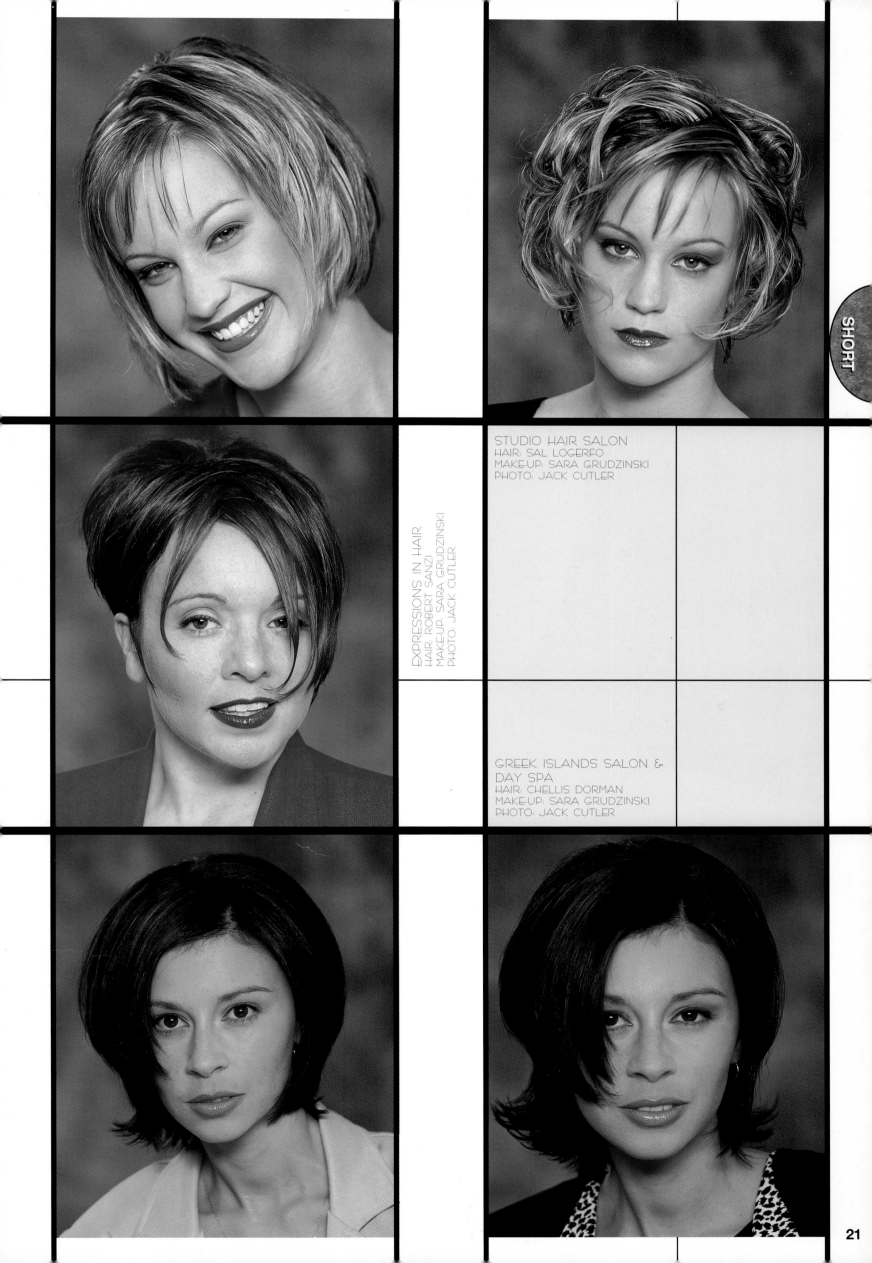

STUDIO HAIR SALON
HAIR: SAL LOGERFO
MAKE-UP: SARA GRUDZINSKI
PHOTO: JACK CUTLER

EXPRESSIONS IN HAIR
HAIR: ROBERT SANZI
MAKE-UP: SARA GRUDZINSKI
PHOTO: JACK CUTLER

GREEK ISLANDS SALON &
DAY SPA
HAIR: CHELLIS DORMAN
MAKE-UP: SARA GRUDZINSKI
PHOTO: JACK CUTLER

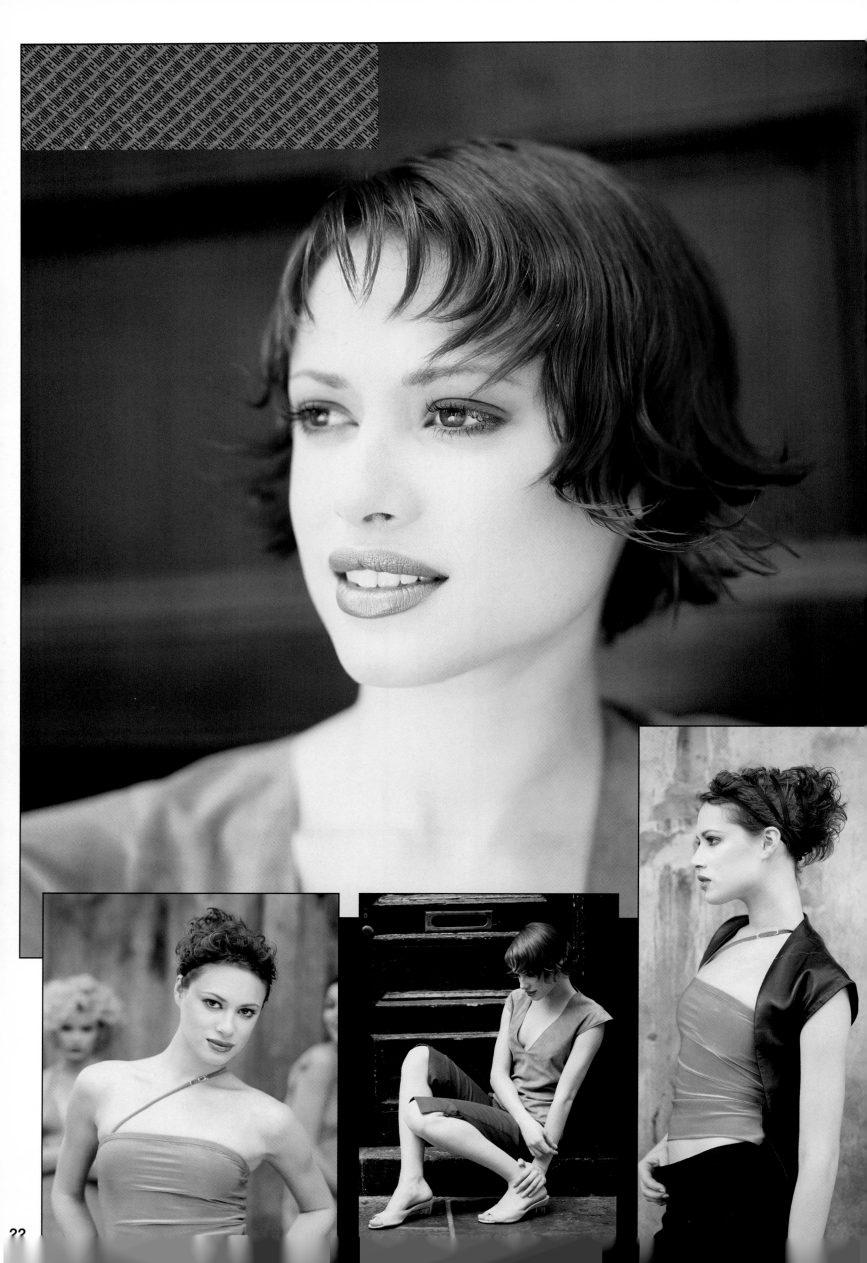

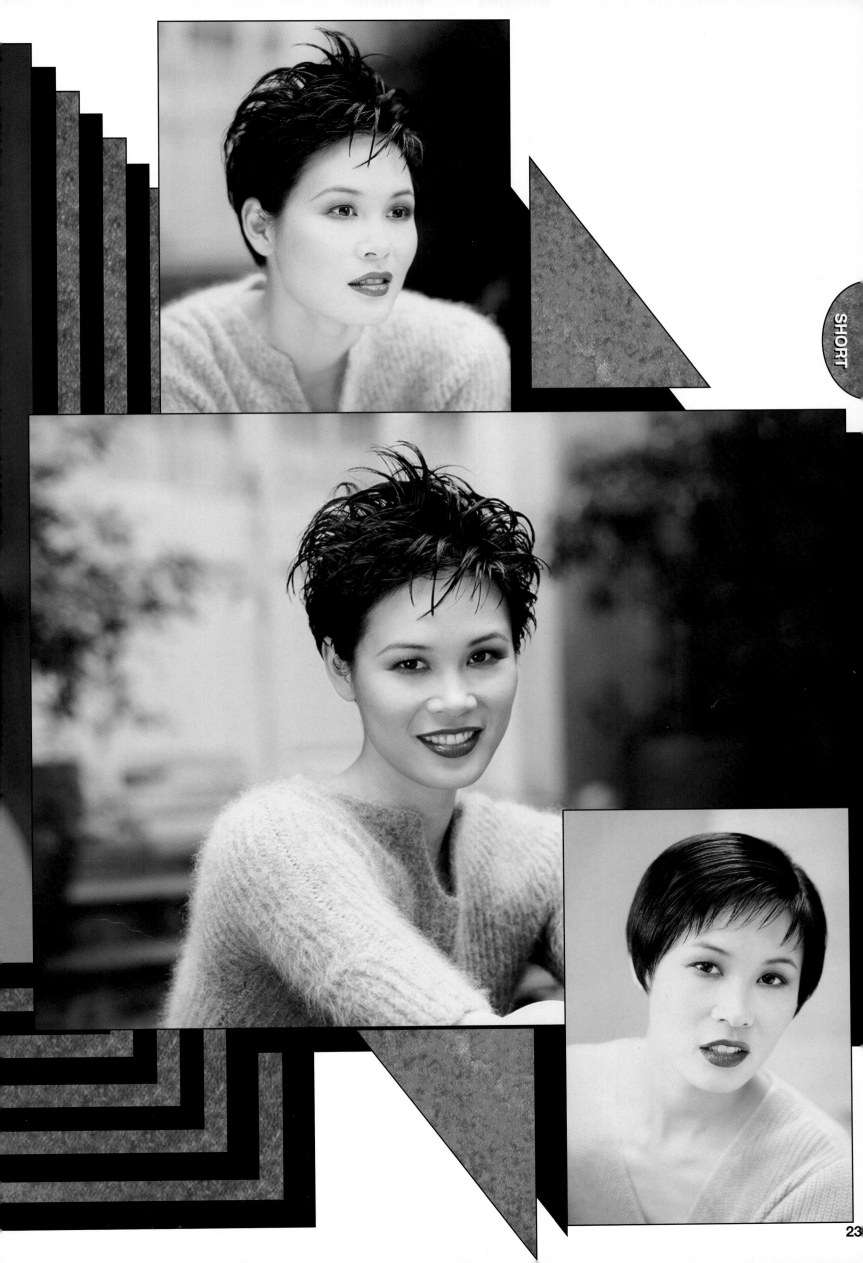

Free flowing mid length layers maintaining a shorter length interior with disconnected panels. Point-cut for extra texture.

Strong rounded fringe with two panels of disconnection on the crown and sides. The back is cut with a rounded layer technique that follows the contour of the head shape.

Robert J. Bushy

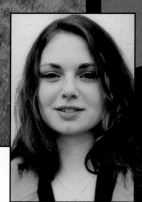

BEFORE

Salon 2000

SALON 2000
HAIR: ROBERT BUSHY
MAKEUP: MICHE NELSON
PHOTO: TOM MCINVAILLE

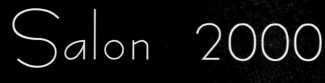

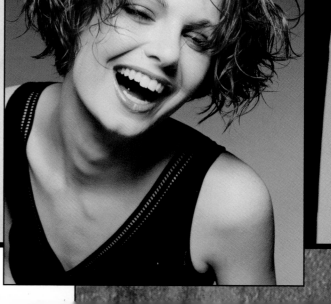

SALON i.d.

HAIR: ERIC GUERIN
PHOTO: SEBASTIAN CIMETTA

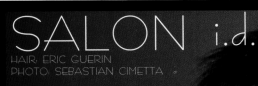

The model's hair was cut short on the side and at the nape. The top was left overlapping the bottom to create more dimension and was texturized for more movement.

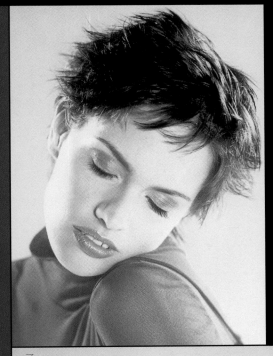

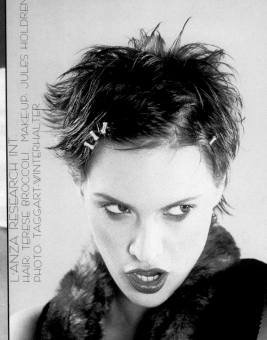

L'ANZA RESEARCH INT.
HAIR: TERESE BROCCOLI MAKEUP: JULES HOLDREN
PHOTO: TAGGART-WINTERHALTER

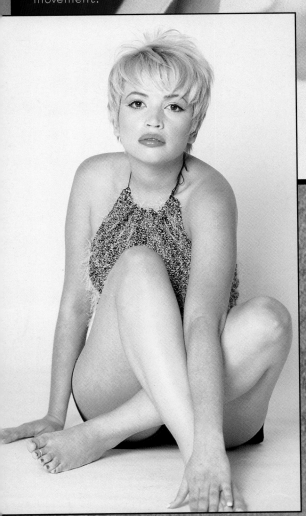

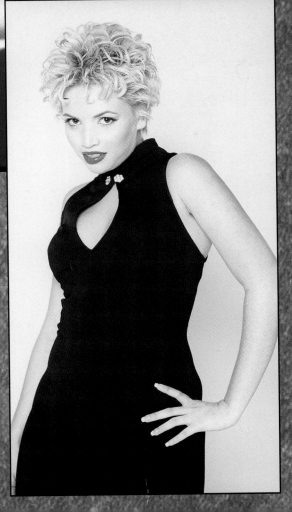

TIMOTHY MARTIN SALON
HAIR: TIMOTHY MARTIN
MAKEUP: MARIA GOMEZ
PHOTO: CORINE SKOTNICA

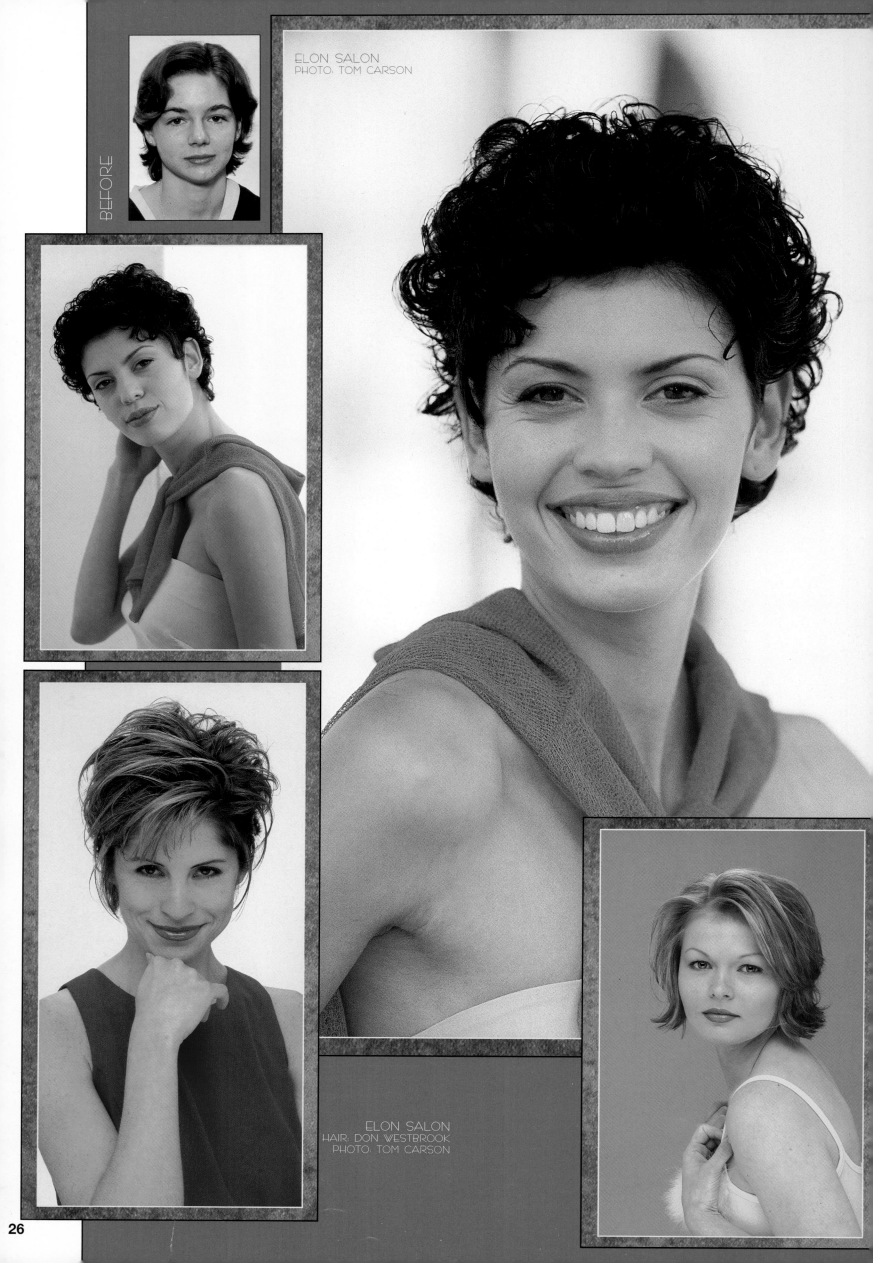

ELON SALON
PHOTO: TOM CARSON

ELON SALON
HAIR: DON WESTBROOK
PHOTO: TOM CARSON

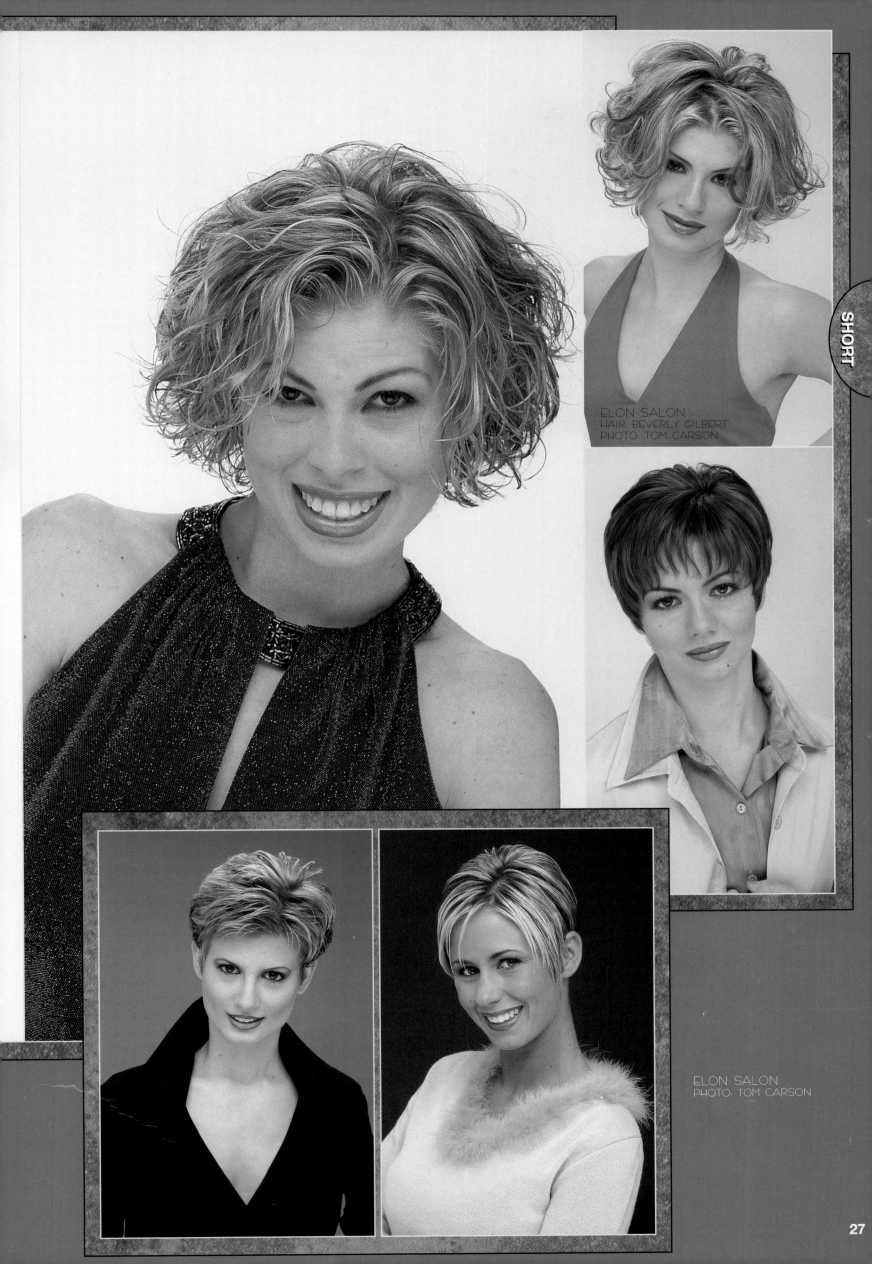

ELON SALON
HAIR: BEVERLY GILBERT
PHOTO: TOM CARSON

ELON SALON
PHOTO: TOM CARSON

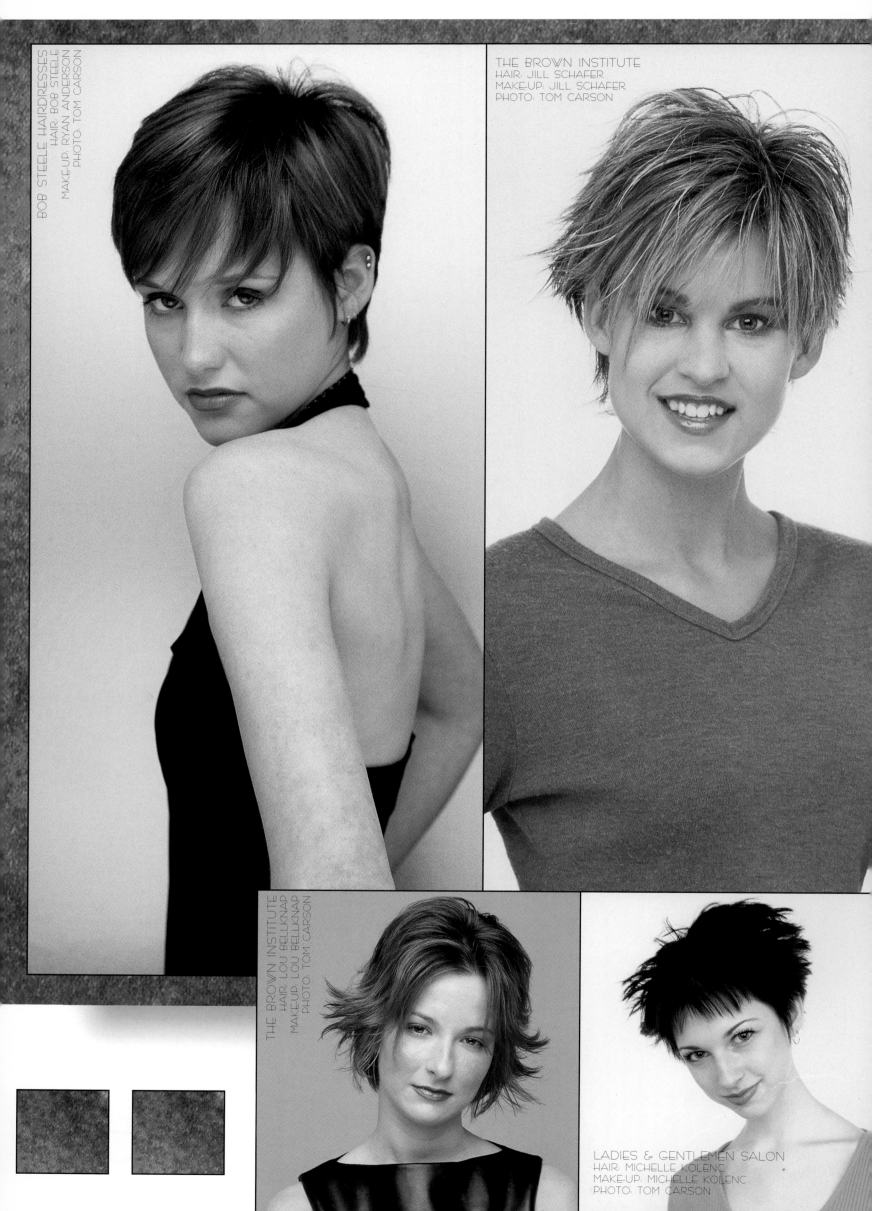

THE BROWN INSTITUTE
HAIR: JILL SCHAFER
MAKE-UP: JILL SCHAFER
PHOTO: TOM CARSON

THE BROWN INSTITUTE
HAIR: LOU BELLKNAP
MAKE-UP: LOU BELLKNAP
PHOTO: TOM CARSON

LADIES & GENTLEMEN SALON
HAIR: MICHELLE KOLENC
MAKE-UP: MICHELLE KOLENC
PHOTO: TOM CARSON

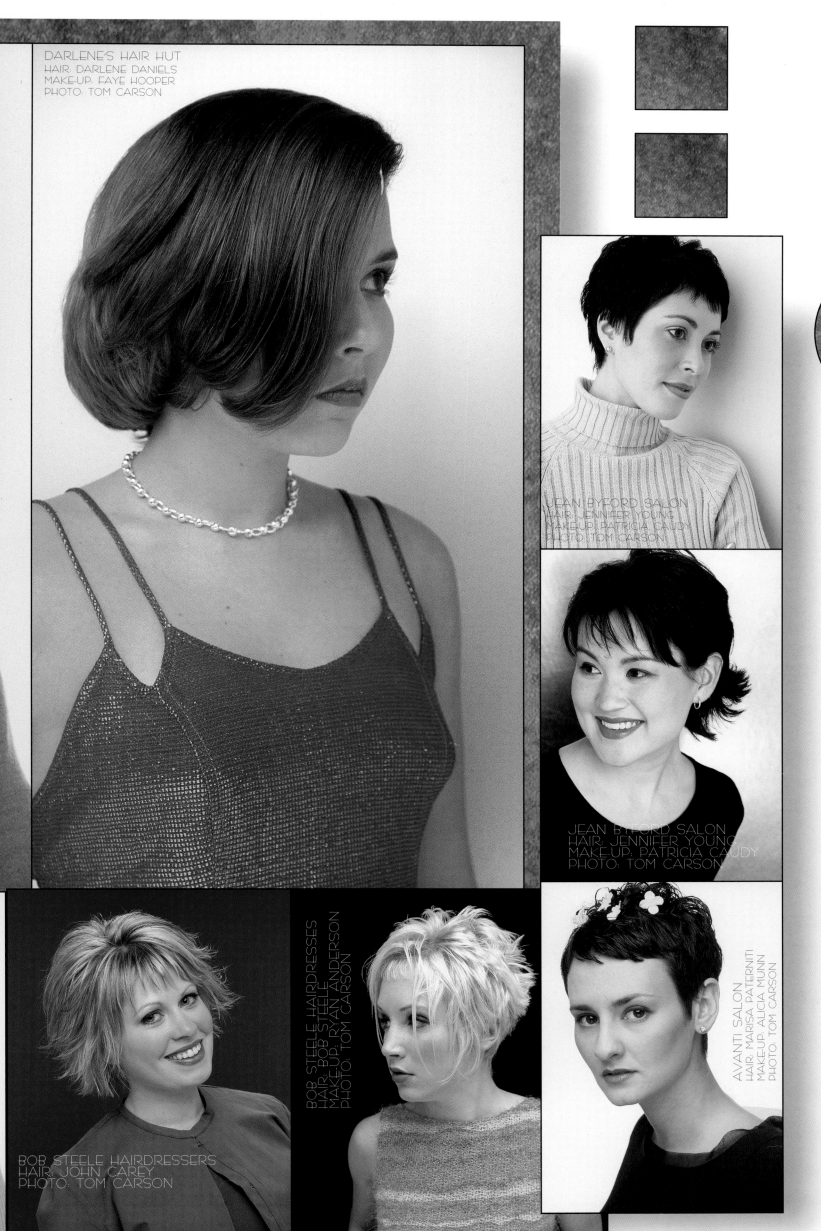

DARLENE'S HAIR HUT
HAIR: DARLENE DANIELS
MAKE-UP: FAYE HOOPER
PHOTO: TOM CARSON

JEAN BYFORD SALON
HAIR: JENNIFER YOUNG
MAKE-UP: PATRICIA CAUDY
PHOTO: TOM CARSON

JEAN BYFORD SALON
HAIR: JENNIFER YOUNG
MAKE-UP: PATRICIA CAUDY
PHOTO: TOM CARSON

BOB STEELE HAIRDRESSERS
HAIR: JOHN CAREY
PHOTO: TOM CARSON

BOB STEELE HAIRDRESSES
HAIR: BOB STEELE
MAKE-UP: RYAN ANDERSON
PHOTO: TOM CARSON

AVANTI SALON
HAIR: MARISA PATERNITI
MAKE-UP: ALICIA MUNN
PHOTO: TOM CARSON

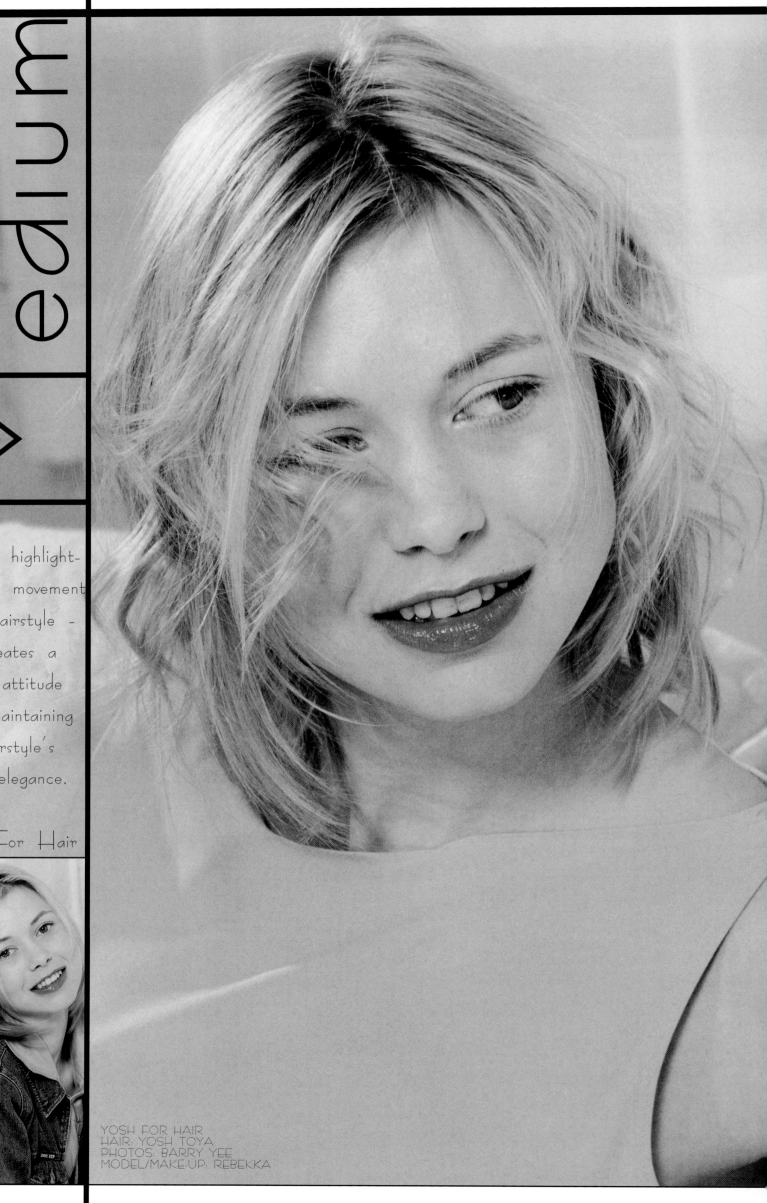

Medium

I enjoy highlighting the movement of a hairstyle - this creates a playful attitude while maintaining the hairstyle's simple elegance.

Yosh For Hair

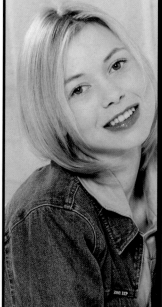

YOSH FOR HAIR
HAIR: YOSH TOYA
PHOTOS: BARRY YEE
MODEL/MAKE-UP: REBEKKA

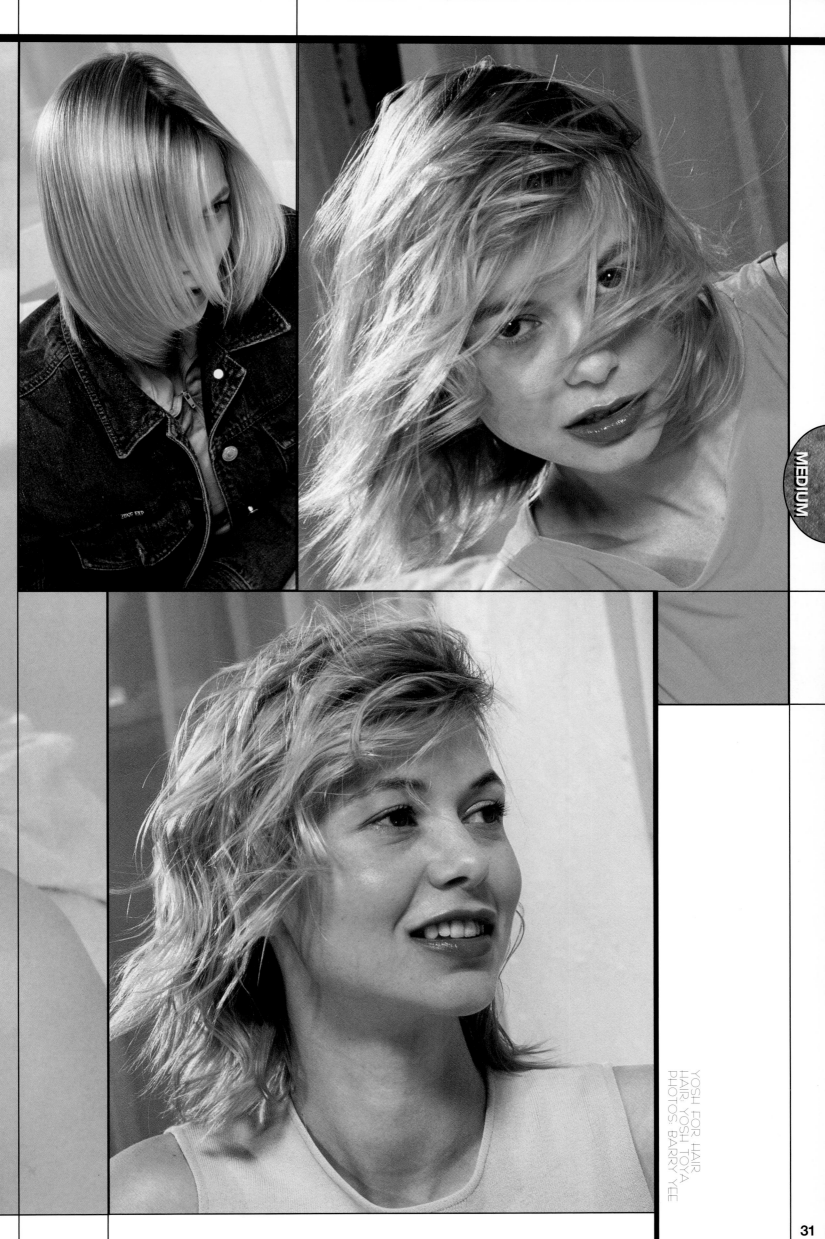

MEDIUM

YOSH FOR HAIR
HAIR: YOSH TOYA
PHOTOS: BARRY YEE

Francesco Group

Celestial –
Versatility.

The mysterious
female form.

FRANCESCO GROUP
HAIR: SHARON PEAKE
MAKE-UP: VANESSA HAINES
PHOTO: PETER DELLICOMPAGNI

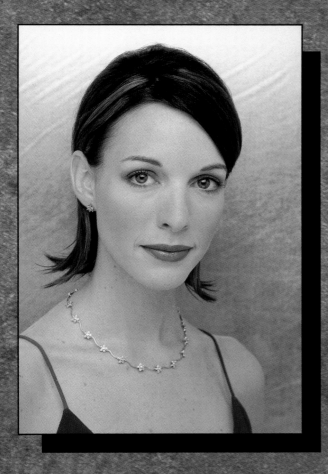

MEDIUM

SALON NEXT
HAIR: TUCKER/ADAM STEWART   MAKE-UP: ROANNA BALES
PHOTO: TOM CARSON

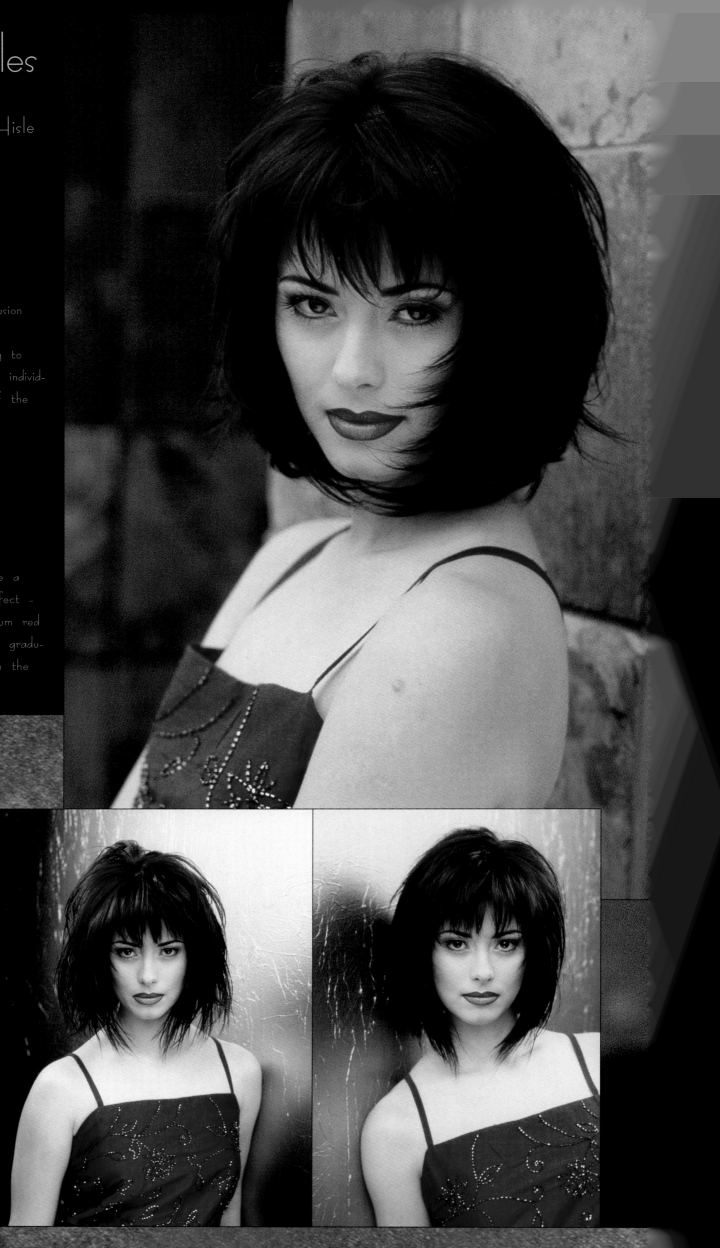

Scruples

Heidemarie Hisle

The Cut:
Intrinsic Razor Fusion

(Intrinsic- pertaining to the essence of the individual... Expression of the real self.

The Color:
Contour Fusion

I wanted to achieve a subtle shadowing effect - going from a medium red color on top, to a graduated darker red on the bottom perimeter.

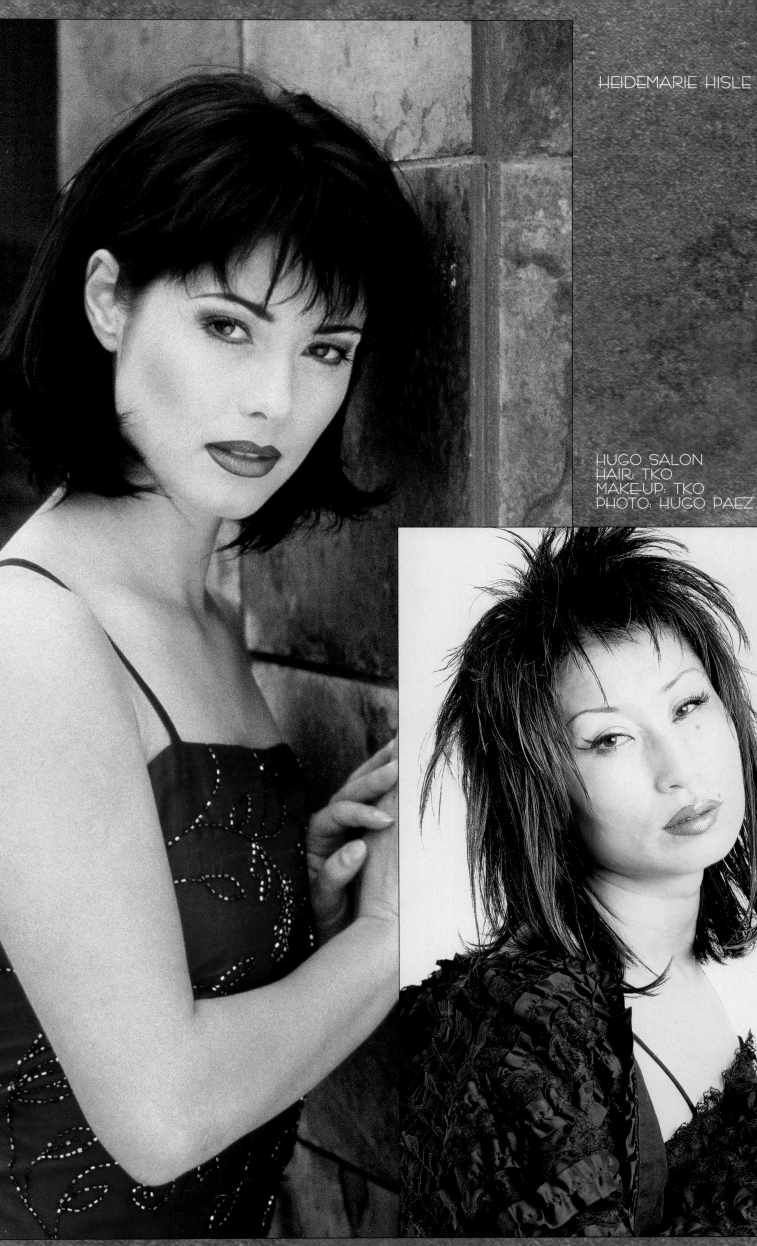

HUGO SALON
HAIR: TKO
MAKEUP: TKO
PHOTO: HUGO PAEZ

MEDIUM

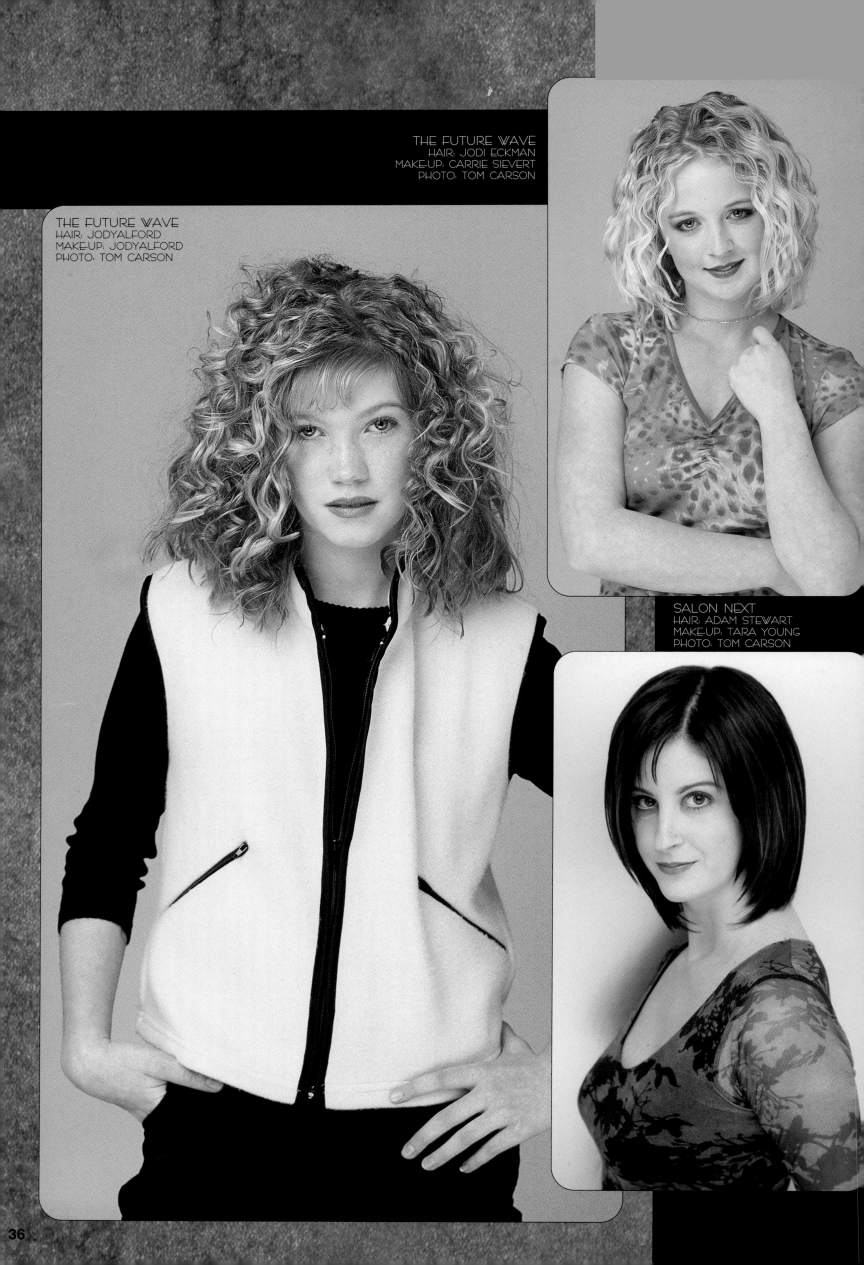

THE FUTURE WAVE
HAIR: JODI ECKMAN
MAKE-UP: CARRIE SIEVERT
PHOTO: TOM CARSON

THE FUTURE WAVE
HAIR: JODYALFORD
MAKE-UP: JODYALFORD
PHOTO: TOM CARSON

SALON NEXT
HAIR: ADAM STEWART
MAKE-UP: TARA YOUNG
PHOTO: TOM CARSON

SALON RED
HAIR: MONIQUE HAYNES/ROBIN KOOHEN
MAKE-UP: STEPHANIE WHEELER
PHOTO: TOM CARSON

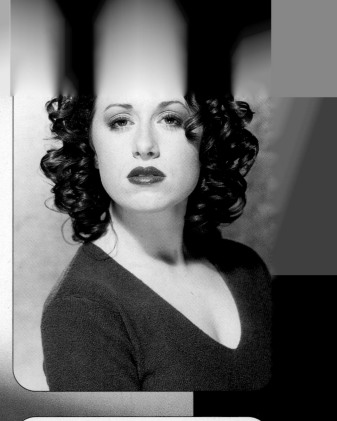

THE BROWN INSTITUTE
HAIR: STEFAIE MESZAROS
MAKE-UP: STEFAIE MESZAROS
PHOTO: TOM CARSON

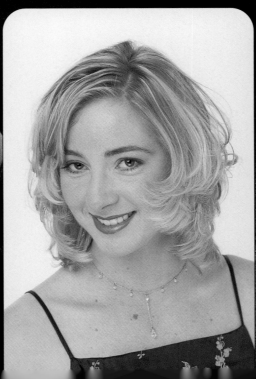

THE FUTURE WAVE SALON
HAIR: MARIE SMOOT MAKE-UP:
MARIE SMOOT
PHOTO: TOM CARSON

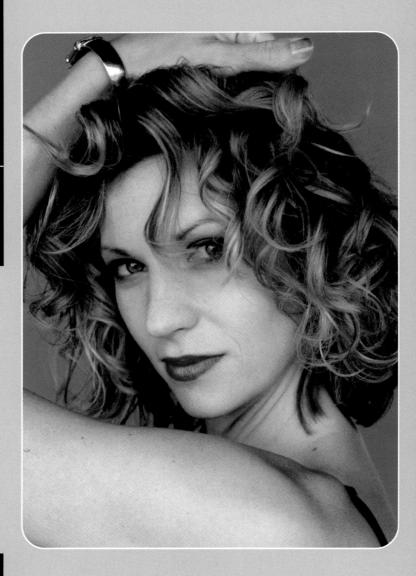

DIZIN SALON
HAIR: BETH ECKEL
PHOTO: BETH ECKEL

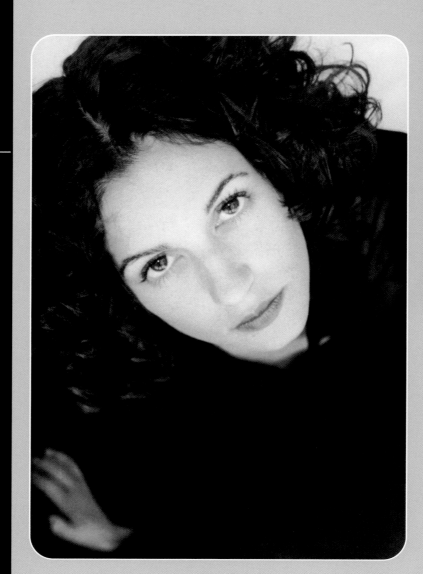

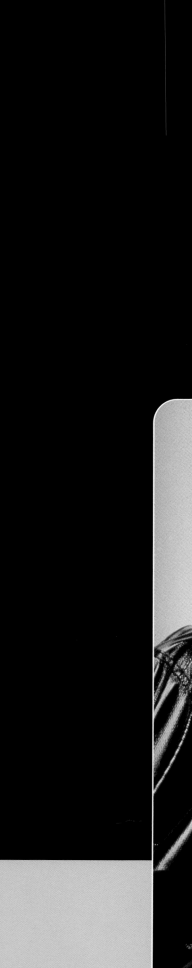

SALON i.d.

HAIR: ERIC GUERIN
PHOTO: SSTIEN CIMETTA

Springy ringlets give this look fabulous texture. The model's curls were perfected with the fingers to make sure the curls were evenly distributed around the head.

Hair was hand painted to add dimension. Amber chestnut and golden blonde colors were used.

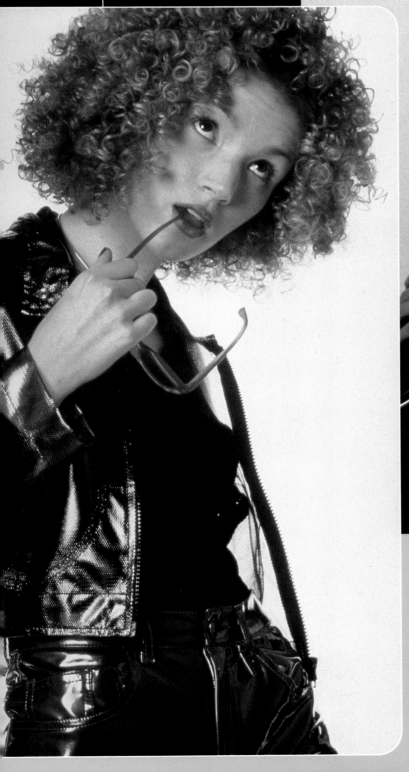

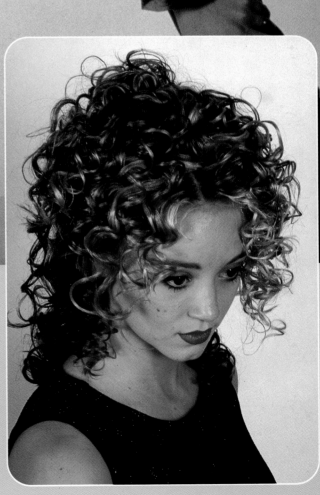

VON CURTIS ACADEMY
HAIR: ANGIE APPLINGTON
MAKE-UP: ANGIE APPLINGTON
PHOTO: DIMITRI HALKIDIS

MEDIUM

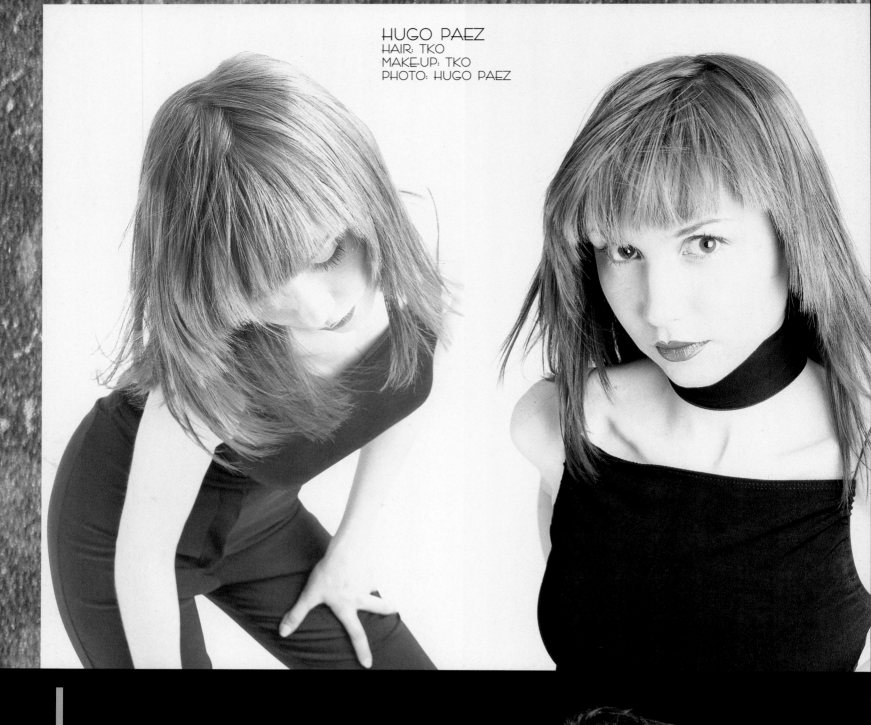

HUGO PAEZ
HAIR: TKO
MAKE-UP: TKO
PHOTO: HUGO PAEZ

Long Hair

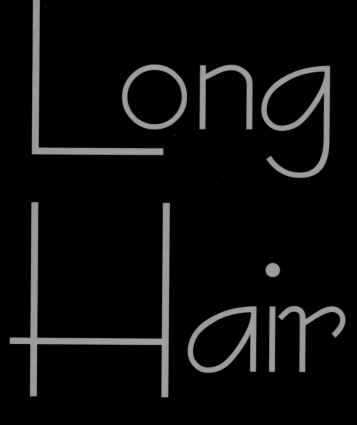

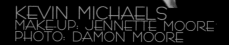

KEVIN MICHAELS
MAKE-UP: JENNETTE MOORE
PHOTO: DAMON MOORE

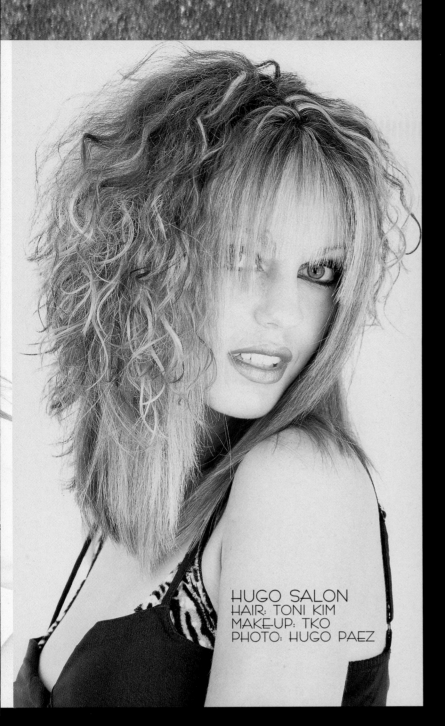

HUGO SALON
HAIR: TONI KIM
MAKE-UP: TKO
PHOTO: HUGO PAEZ

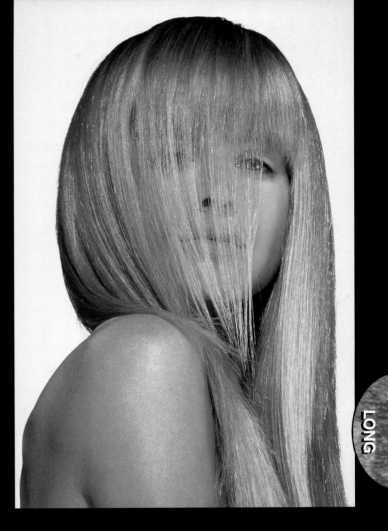

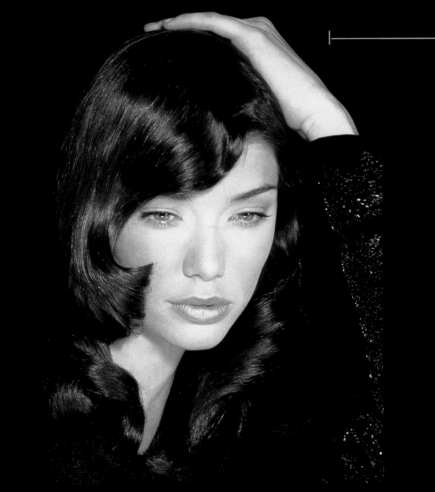

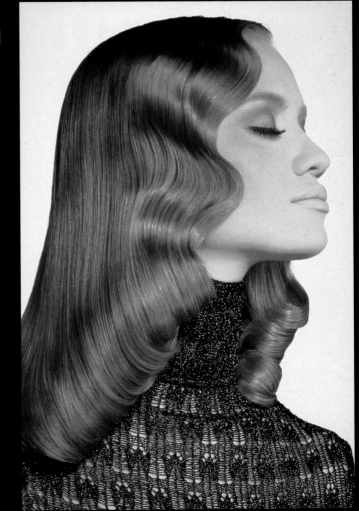

KEVIN MICHAELS
MAKEUP: JENNETTE MOORE
PHOTO: DAMON MOORE

L'IMAGE SALONS
HAIR DAYTON MAST
PHOTO: D. MAST

L'Image Salon:

Romance Revisited

Turn up the heat this fall with beautiful blonde highlights and romantic curls. Thick loopy curls were achieved by sectioning the hair and placing a curling iron at the root. Remaining hair was then wrapped downward around the curling iron.

Dayton Mast

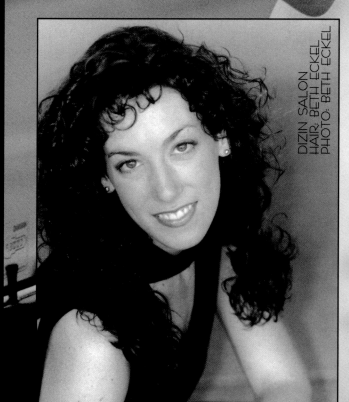

DIZIN SALON
HAIR: BETH ECKEL
PHOTO: BETH ECKEL

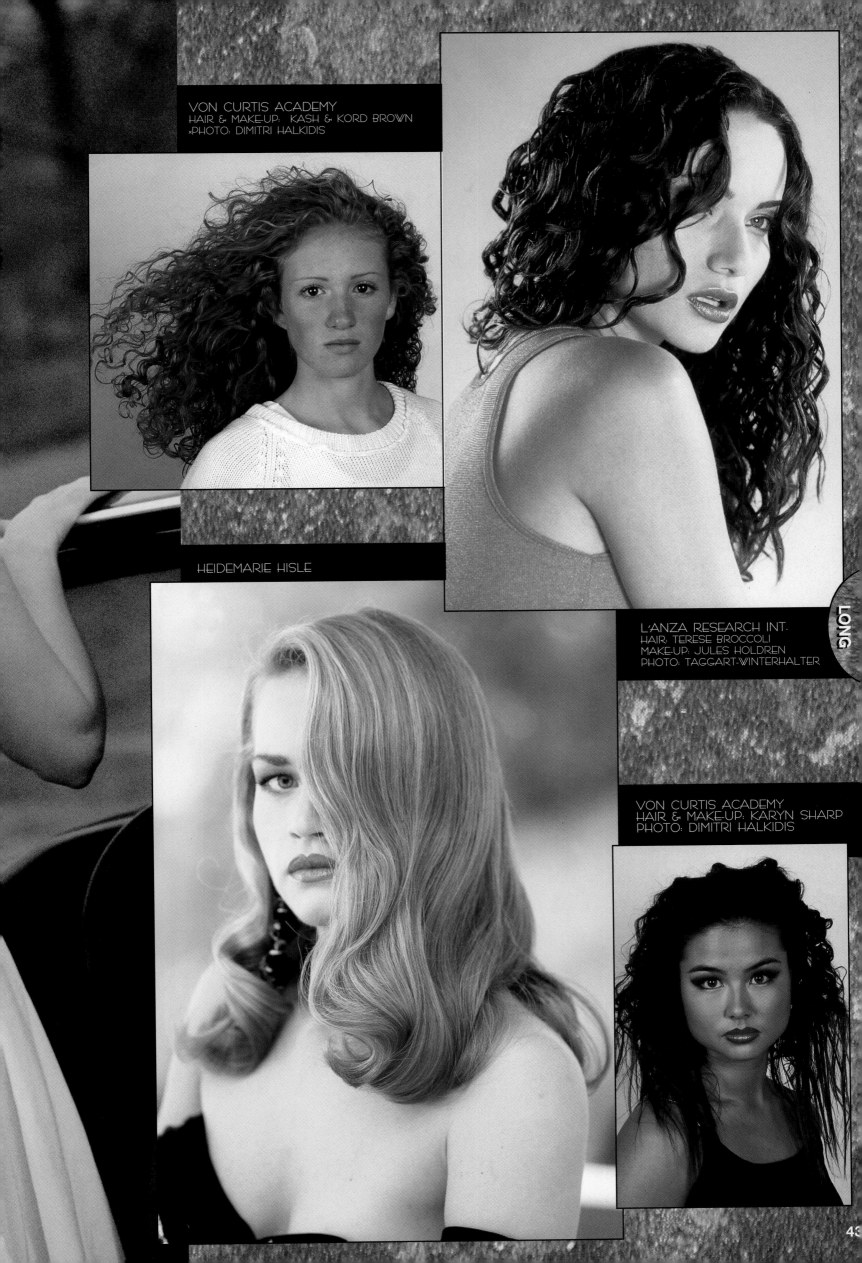

VON CURTIS ACADEMY
HAIR & MAKE-UP: KASH & KORD BROWN
*PHOTO: DIMITRI HALKIDIS

HEIDEMARIE HISLE

L'ANZA RESEARCH INT.
HAIR: TERESE BROCCOLI
MAKE-UP: JULES HOLDREN
PHOTO: TAGGART-WINTERHALTER

VON CURTIS ACADEMY
HAIR & MAKE-UP: KARYN SHARP
PHOTO: DIMITRI HALKIDIS

LONG

43

Gene Jaurez

Long hair is feminine, soft and sensual, with untamed locks.

Subtle layers were added to build in more texture and volume.

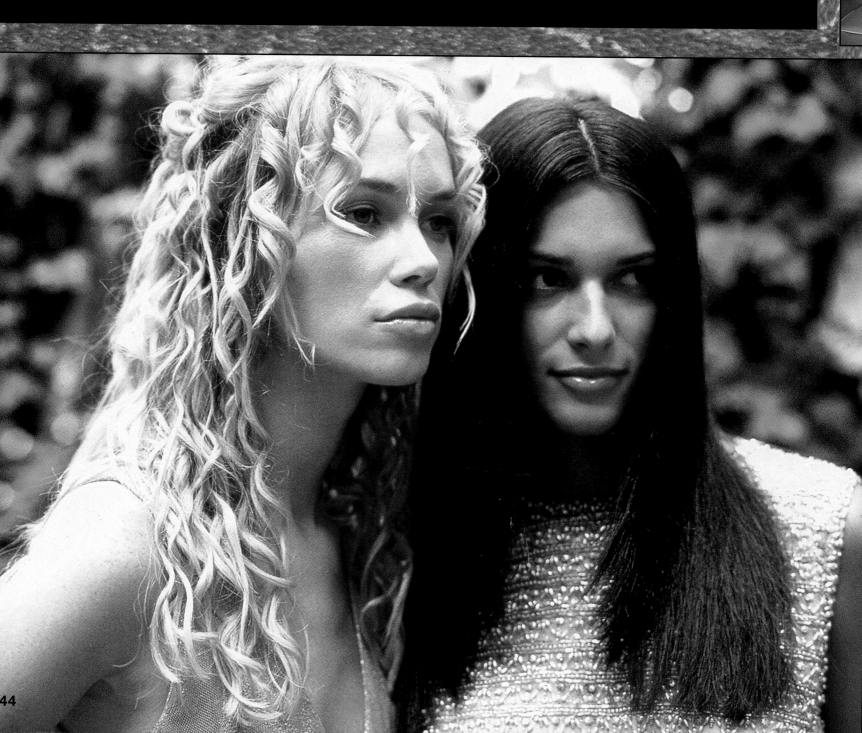

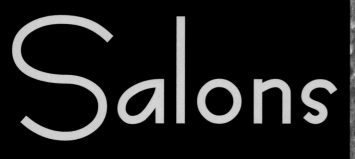

Salons

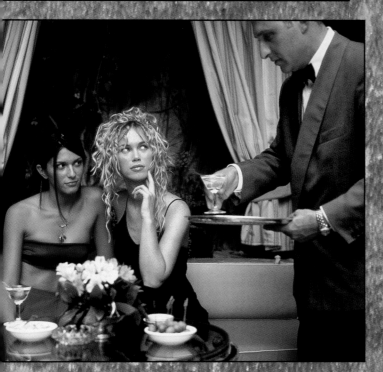

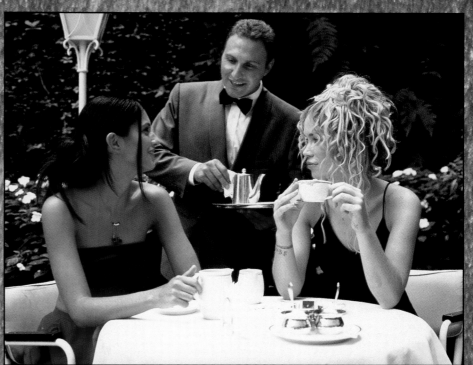

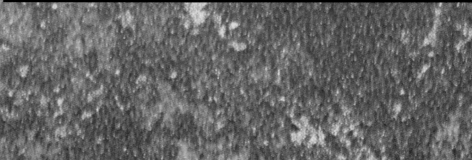

GENE JUAREZ SALON
HAIR: GENE JUAREZ SALON ARTISTS   MAKE-UP: TIZIANA   PHOTO: SVEVA BELLUCCI

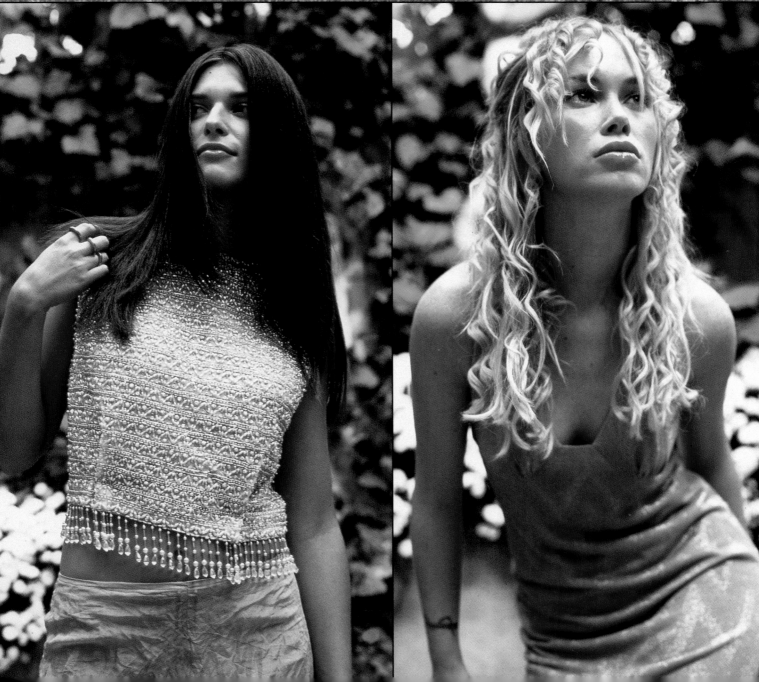

LONG

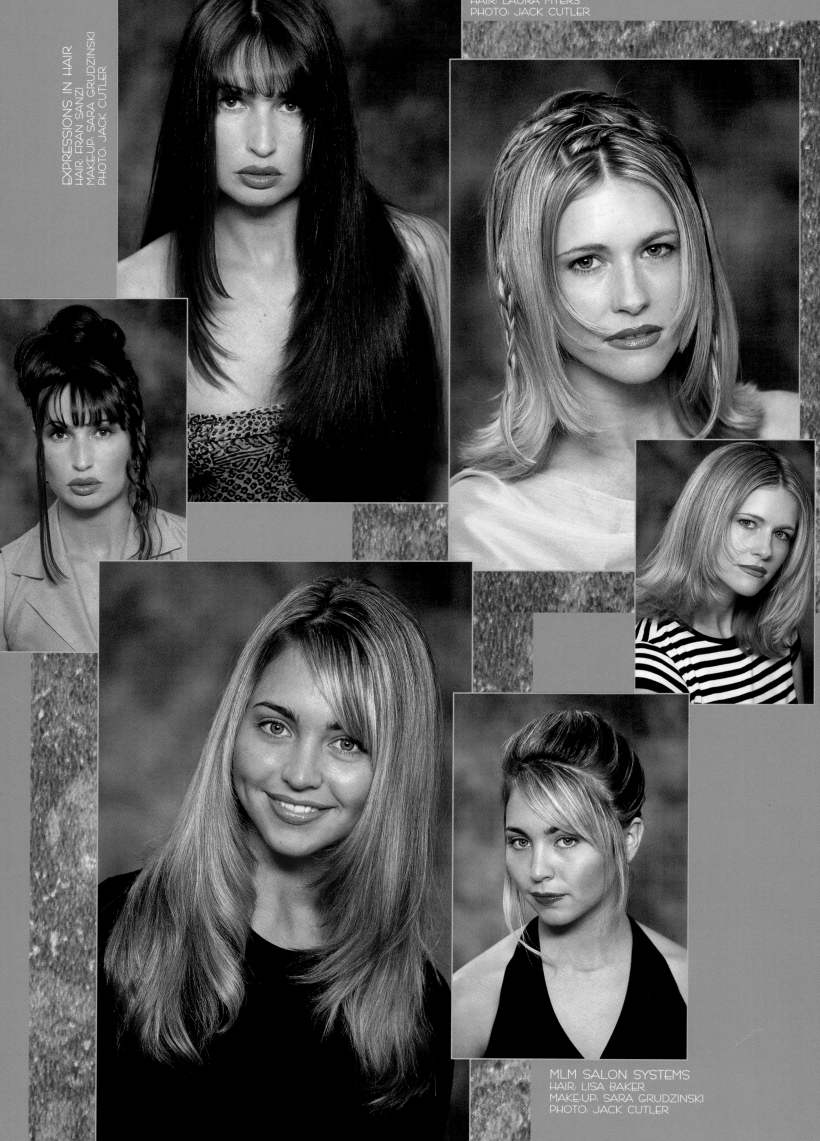

EXPRESSIONS IN HAIR
HAIR: FRAN SANZI
MAKEUP: SARA GRUDZINSKI
PHOTO: JACK CUTLER

SCULPTURED IMAGES DAY SPA
HAIR: LAURA MYERS
PHOTO: JACK CUTLER

MLM SALON SYSTEMS
HAIR: LISA BAKER
MAKE-UP: SARA GRUDZINSKI
PHOTO: JACK CUTLER

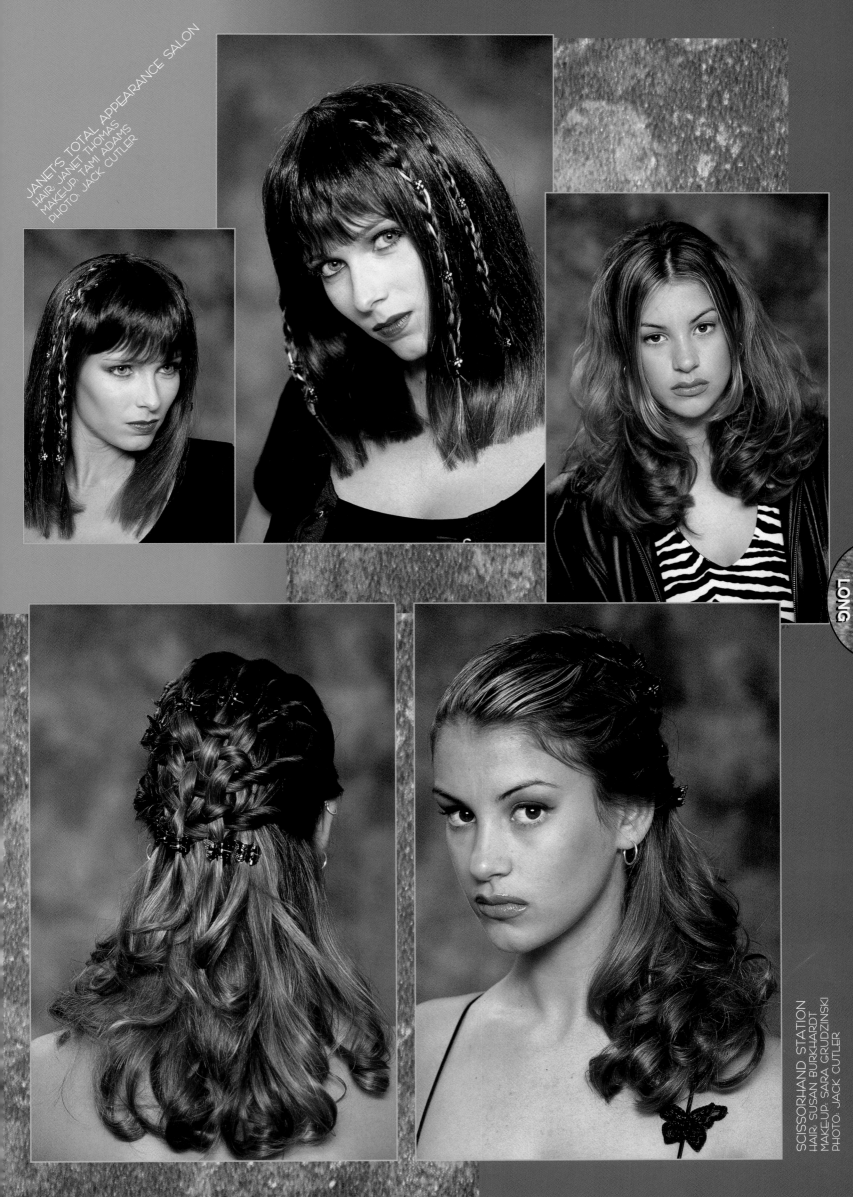

LONG

SCISSORHAND STATION
HAIR: SUSAN BURKHARDT
MAKEUP: SARA GRUDZINSKI
PHOTO: JACK CUTLER

47

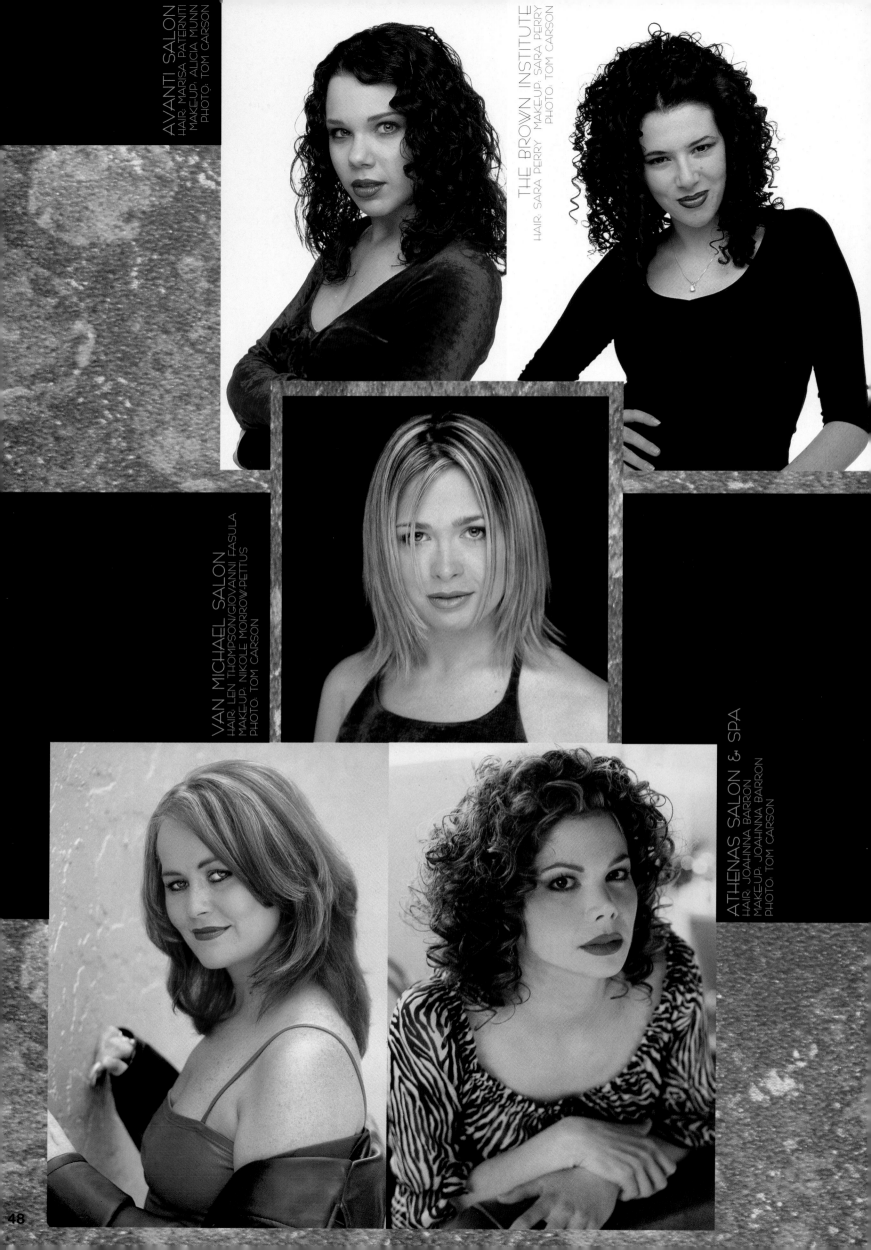

AVANTI SALON
HAIR: MARISA PATERNITI
MAKEUP: ALICIA MUNN
PHOTO: TOM CARSON

THE BROWN INSTITUTE
HAIR: SARA PERRY MAKEUP: SARA PERRY
PHOTO: TOM CARSON

VAN MICHAEL SALON
HAIR: LEN THOMPSON/GIOVANNI FASULA
MAKEUP: NIKOLE MORROW-PETTUS
PHOTO: TOM CARSON

ATHENAS SALON & SPA
HAIR: JOAHNNA BARRON
MAKEUP: JOAHNNA BARRON
PHOTO: TOM CARSON

LADIES & GENTLEMEN SALON
HAIR: LAURA WASHOCK MAKE-UP: LAURA WASHOCK PHOTO: TOM CARSON

DARLENE'S HAIR
HUT
HAIR: DARLENE
DANIELS
MAKE-UP: FAYE
HOOPER
PHOTO:
TOM CARSON

LONG

ATHENAS SALON & SPA
HAIR: JOAHNNA BARRON
MAKE-UP: JOAHNNA BARRON
PHOTO: TOM CARSON

COBALT SALON
HAIR: BERT ROBERTS
MAKE-UP: K.D. ALSADEG
PHOTO: TOM CARSON

49

TEENS

D'aversa
The Salon

Cutting edge,
makeover madness

... teens define
the trends for
their generation.

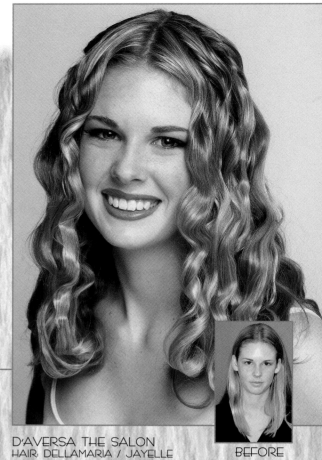

D'AVERSA THE SALON
HAIR: DELLAMARIA / JAYELLE
MAKE-UP: JACQUELINE SHERLOCK
PHOTO: TAGGART-WINTERHALTER

BEFORE

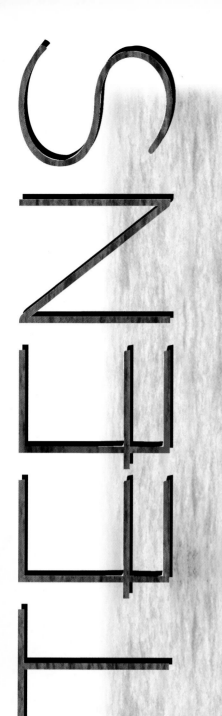

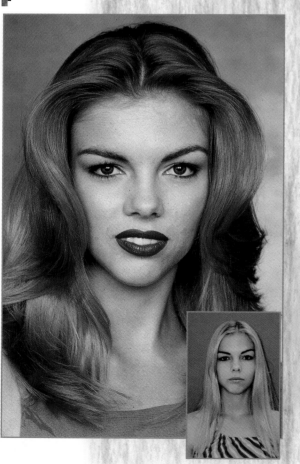

BEFORE

BEFORE

D'AVERSA THE SALON
HAIR: DELLAMARIA / JAYELLE
MAKE-UP: JACQUELINE SHERLOCK
PHOTO: TAGGART WINTERHALTER

BEFORE

ELON SALON
PHOTO: TOM CARSON

BEFORE

Kenneth's Haircutting Inc

This cut and color were created together with texture, texture, and more texture in mind. The dramatic contrast of golden blonde tones compliment the lines in this disconnected razor cut like nothing subtle could.

This trendy style is all about having fun!

KENNETH'S HAIRCUTTING
HAIR: KELLY KIEF
MAKE-UP: MONICA KIEF
PHOTO: JILL COLLOPY

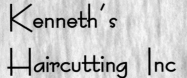

BEFORE

TEENS

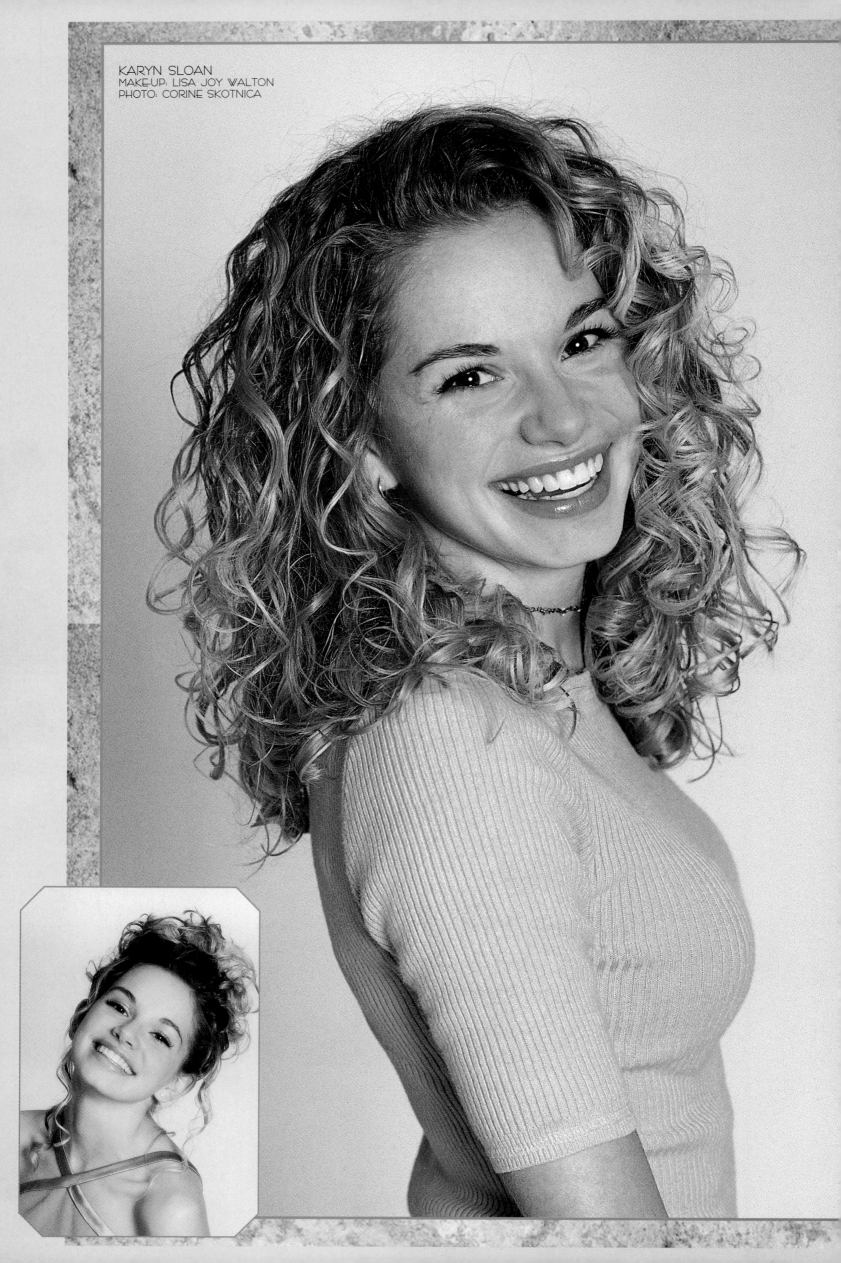

KARYN SLOAN
MAKEUP: LISA JOY WALTON
PHOTO: CORINE SKOTNICA

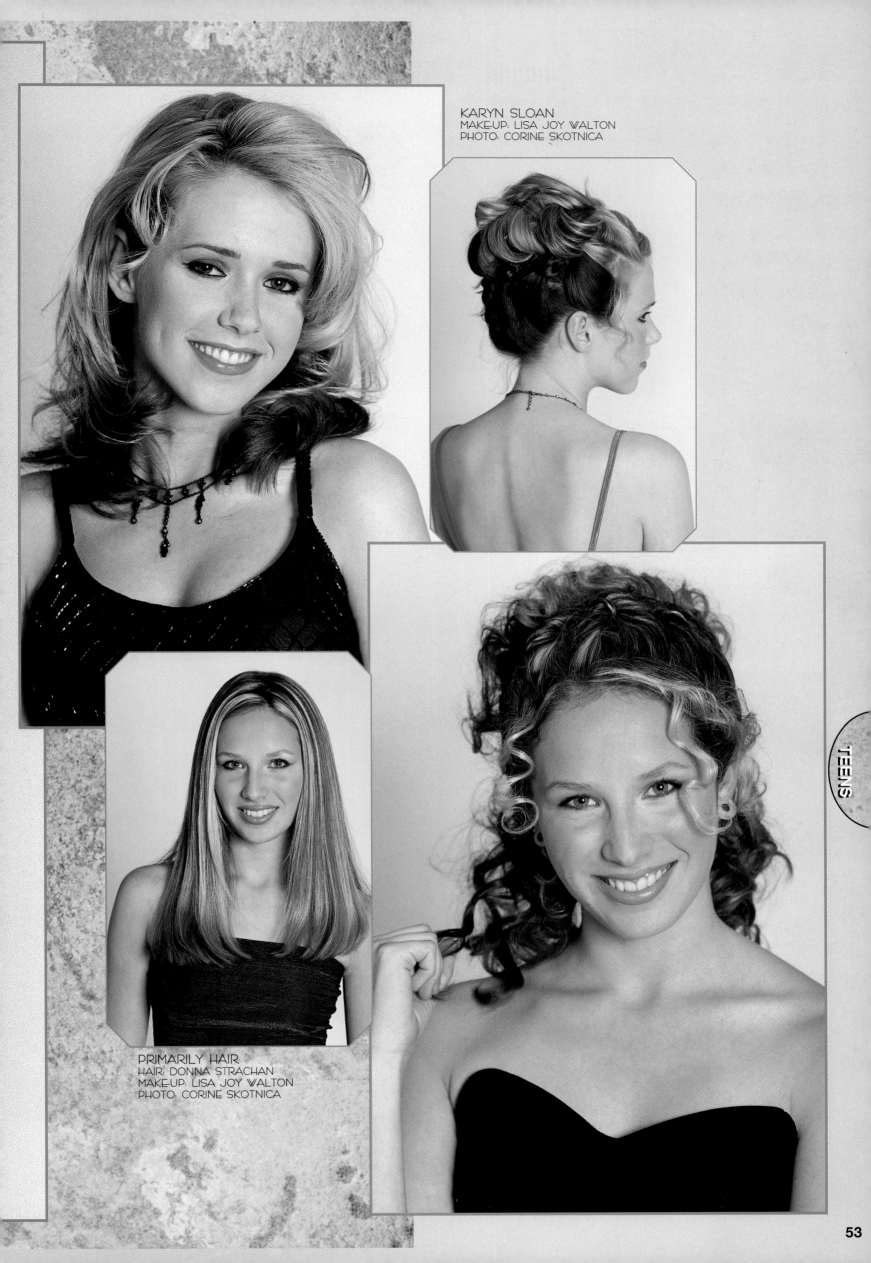

KARYN SLOAN
MAKE-UP: LISA JOY WALTON
PHOTO: CORINE SKOTNICA

PRIMARILY HAIR
HAIR: DONNA STRACHAN
MAKE-UP: LISA JOY WALTON
PHOTO: CORINE SKOTNICA

TEENS

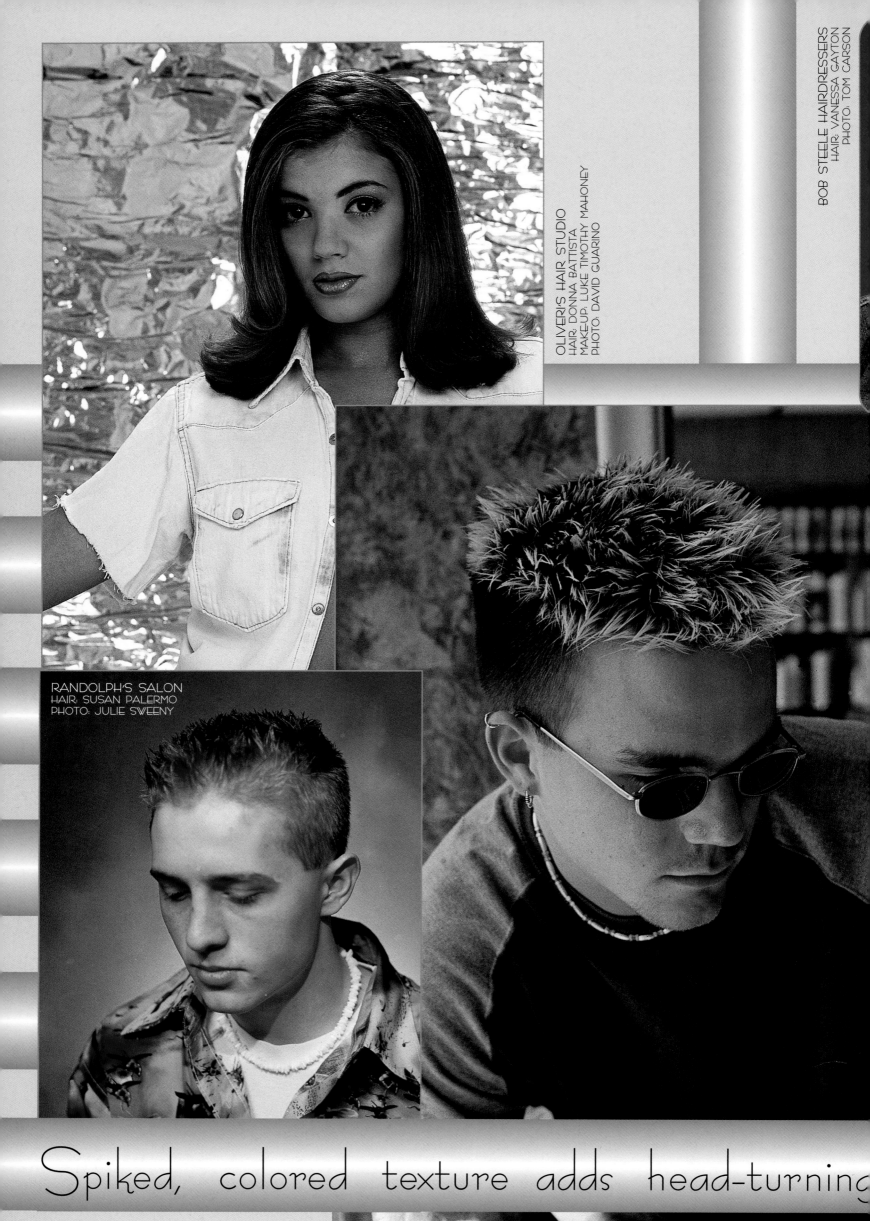

OLIVERI'S HAIR STUDIO
HAIR: DONNA BATTISTA
MAKE-UP: LUKE TIMOTHY MAHONEY
PHOTO: DAVID GUARINO

BOB STEELE HAIRDRESSERS
HAIR: VANESSA GAYTON
PHOTO: TOM CARSON

RANDOLPH'S SALON
HAIR: SUSAN PALERMO
PHOTO: JULIE SWEENY

Spiked, colored texture adds head-turning

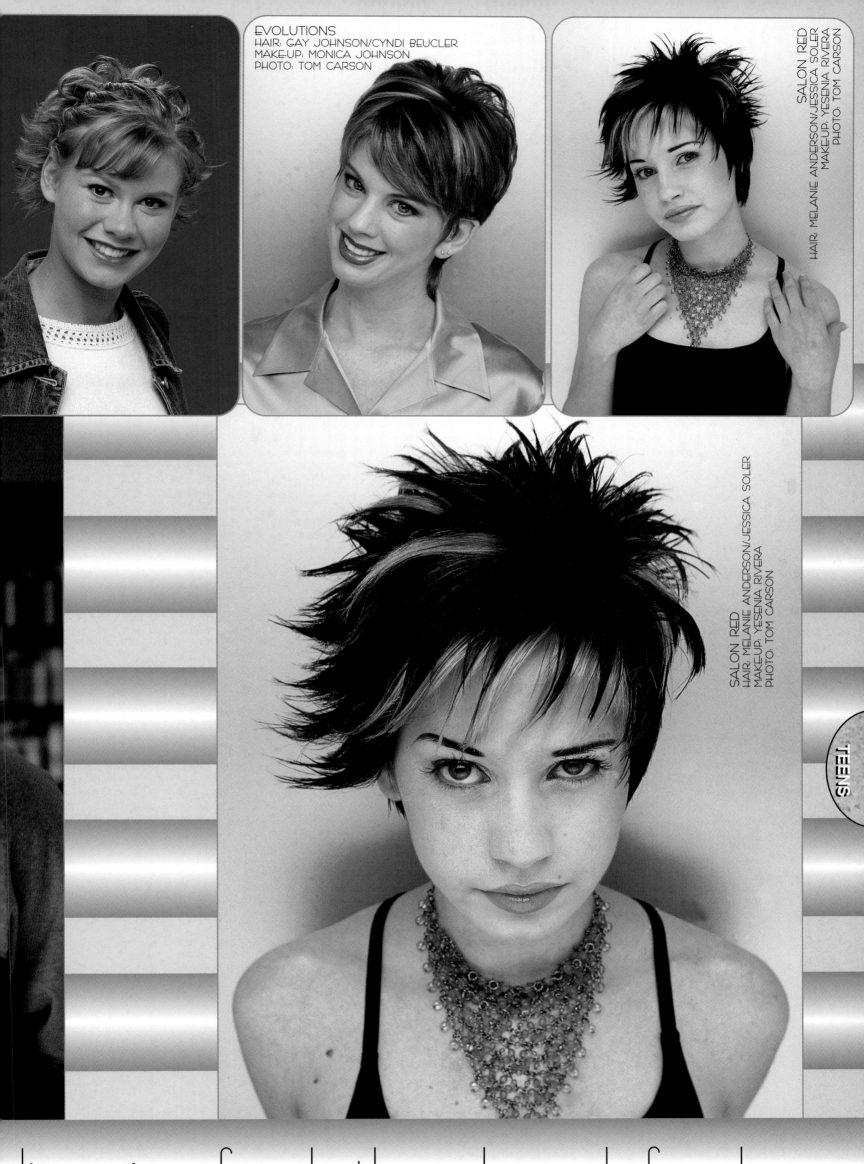

EVOLUTIONS
HAIR: GAY JOHNSON/CYNDI BEUCLER
MAKE-UP: MONICA JOHNSON
PHOTO: TOM CARSON

SALON RED
HAIR: MELANIE ANDERSON/JESSICA SOLER
MAKE-UP: YESENIA RIVERA
PHOTO: TOM CARSON

SALON RED
HAIR: MELANIE ANDERSON/JESSICA SOLER
MAKE-UP: YESENIA RIVERA
PHOTO: TOM CARSON

TEENS

dimension for both male and females.

55

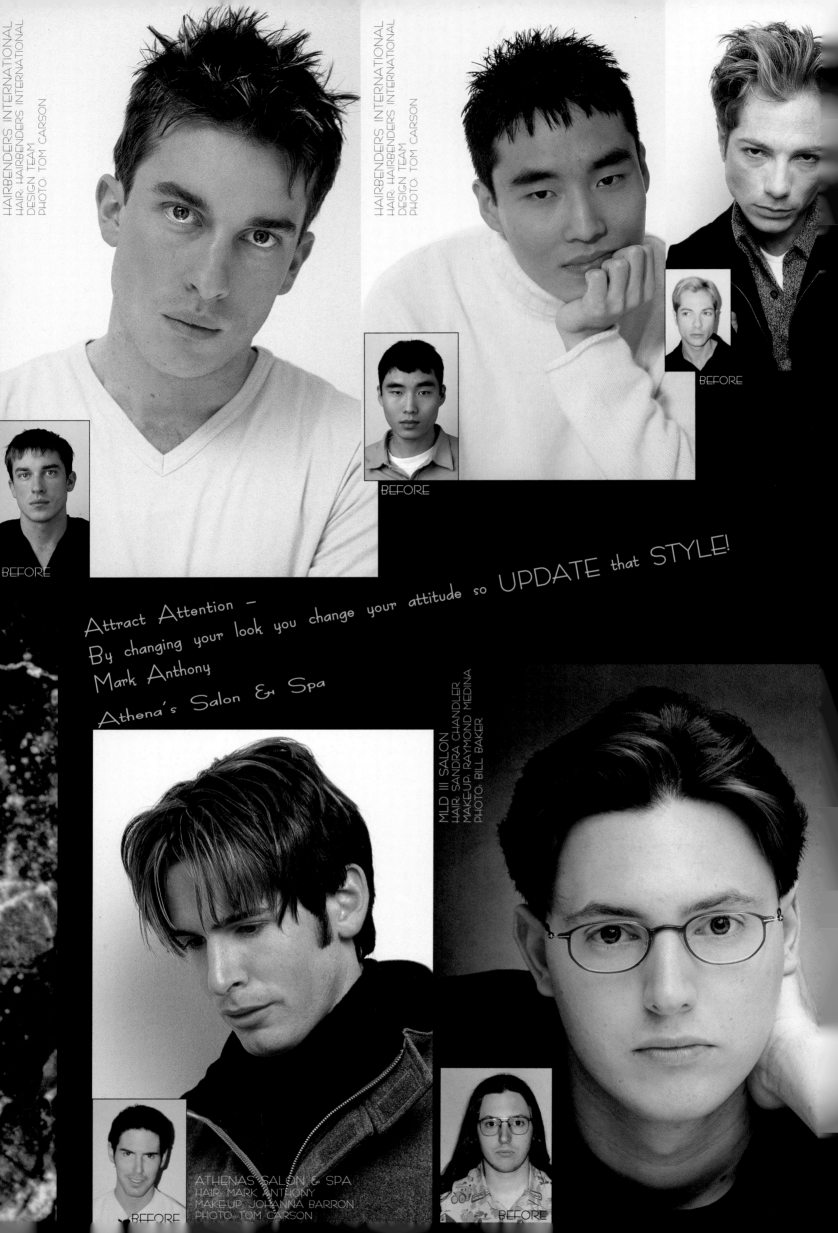

HAIRBENDERS INTERNATIONAL
HAIR: HAIRBENDERS INTERNATIONAL
DESIGN TEAM
PHOTO: TOM CARSON

HAIRBENDERS INTERNATIONAL
HAIR: HAIRBENDERS INTERNATIONAL
DESIGN TEAM
PHOTO: TOM CARSON

BEFORE

BEFORE

BEFORE

Attract Attention —
By changing your look you change your attitude so UPDATE that STYLE!
Mark Anthony
Athena's Salon & Spa

MLD III SALON
HAIR: SANDRA CHANDLER
MAKEUP: RAYMOND MEDINA
PHOTO: BILL BAKER

BEFORE

ATHENAS SALON & SPA
HAIR: MARK ANTHONY
MAKEUP: JOHANNA BARRON
PHOTO: TOM CARSON

BEFORE

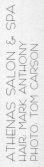

ATHENA'S SALON & SPA
HAIR: MARK ANTHONY
PHOTO: TOM CARSON

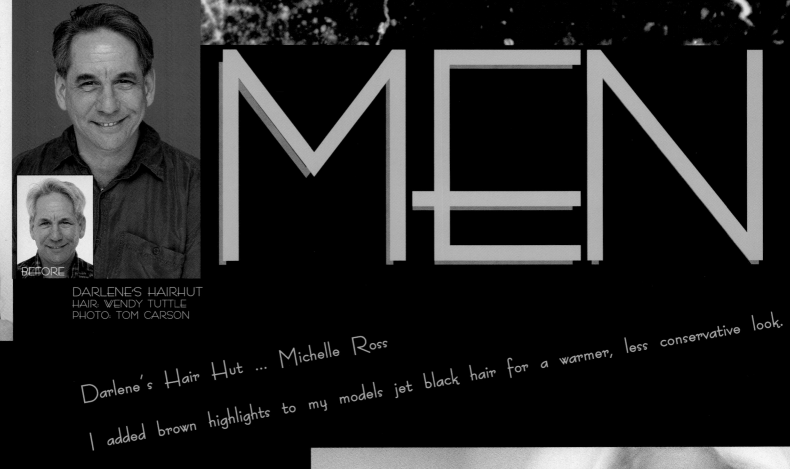

MEN

BEFORE

DARLENE'S HAIRHUT
HAIR: WENDY TUTTLE
PHOTO: TOM CARSON

Darlene's Hair Hut ... Michelle Ross

I added brown highlights to my models jet black hair for a warmer, less conservative look.

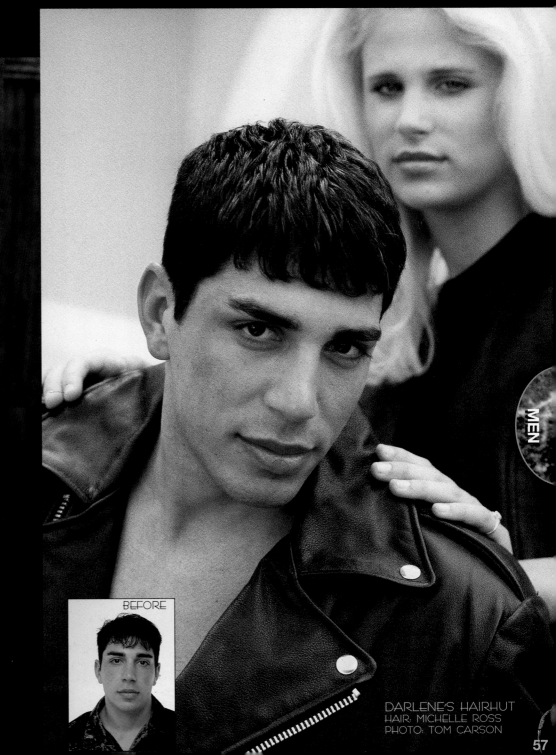

MEN

BEFORE

DARLENE'S HAIRHUT
HAIR: DANA SNOW
PHOTO: TOM CARSON

BEFORE

DARLENE'S HAIRHUT
HAIR: MICHELLE ROSS
PHOTO: TOM CARSON

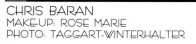

CHRIS BARAN
MAKE-UP: ROSE MARIE
PHOTO: TAGGART-WINTERHALTER

Cobolt Salon ———————
This client needed a more versatile
look. Highlights and a new cut
gave him a younger look that's
trendy and versatile.
Bert Roberts

COBALT SALON
HAIR: BERT ROBERTS
MAKE-UP: STAR HERR
PHOTO: TOM CARSON

LADIES & GENTLEMEN SALON
HAIR: JENNIFER MARKELL
PHOTO: TOM CARSON

VON CURTIS ACADEMY
HAIR: CASSIDY LOWE
MAKE-UP: CASSIDY LOWE
PHOTO: MARC REYNOLDS

Evolutions Hair Designs

Highlights were added to
update this conservative
lawyer's look.
Jay Johnson

MLD III SALON
HAIR: SANDRA CHANDLER
MAKE-UP: RAYMOND MEDINA
PHOTO: BILL BAKER

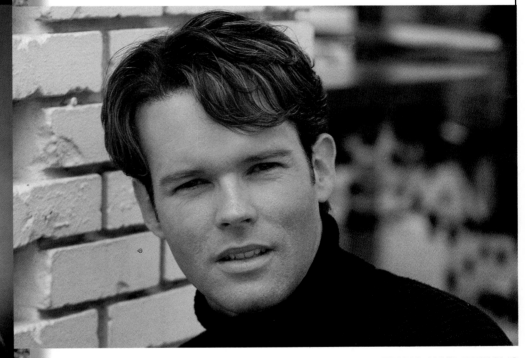

EVOLUTIONS HAIR DESIGNS
HAIR: JAY JOHNSON & CINDY BEUCLER
MAKE-UP: MONICA JOHNSON
PHOTO: TOM CARSON

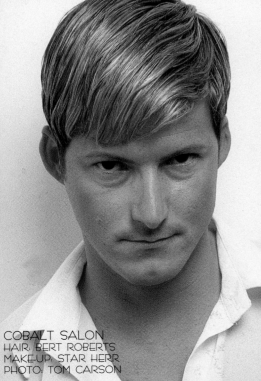

COBALT SALON
HAIR: BERT ROBERTS
MAKE-UP: STAR HERR
PHOTO: TOM CARSON

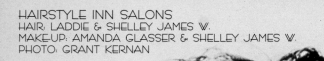

HAIRSTYLE INN SALONS
HAIR: LADDIE & SHELLEY JAMES W.
MAKE-UP: AMANDA GLASSER & SHELLEY JAMES W.
PHOTO: GRANT KERNAN

DIZIN SALON
HAIR: BETH ECKEL
PHOTO: BETH ECKEL

CALISTA GRAND
HAIR: SHERI COWAN
MAKE-UP: DAWN OGDEN
PHOTO: JODY MISTECKA

MLD III SALON
HAIR: SANDRA CHANDLER
MAKEUP: RAYMOND MEDINA
PHOTO: BILL BAKER

RINALDO'S HAIR SALON LLC
HAIR: RINALDO DICIOCCIO
MAKEUP: NICOLE CASSARINO
PHOTO: PHOTO PROS STUDIO

COMPANY HAIR
HAIR: COMPANY HAIR ARTISTIC TEAM
PHOTO: DERMOT MCGIVERN

MEN

61

OVER 30

This cut and color match the model's personality perfectly. A short and sassy hairstyle that's easy to maintain with nothing more than finger drying is Kenneth's signature.

The color is alive with bright highlights that give a little bit of drama to the coppery red.

RANDOLPH'S SALON
HAIR: SCOTT RANDOLPH
PHOTO: JULIE SWEENY

KENNETH'S HAIRCUTTING
HAIR: KENNETH COLLOPY
PHOTO: JILL COLLOPY

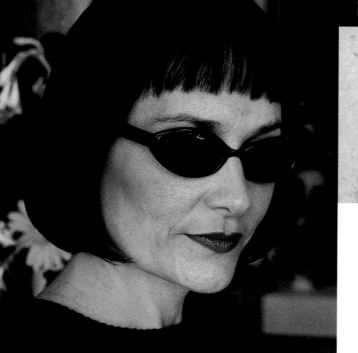

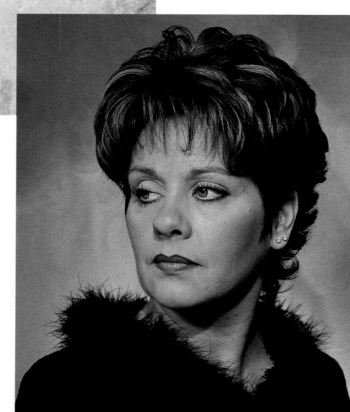

RANDOLPH'S SALON
HAIR: SUSAN PALERMO
PHOTO: JULIE SWEENY

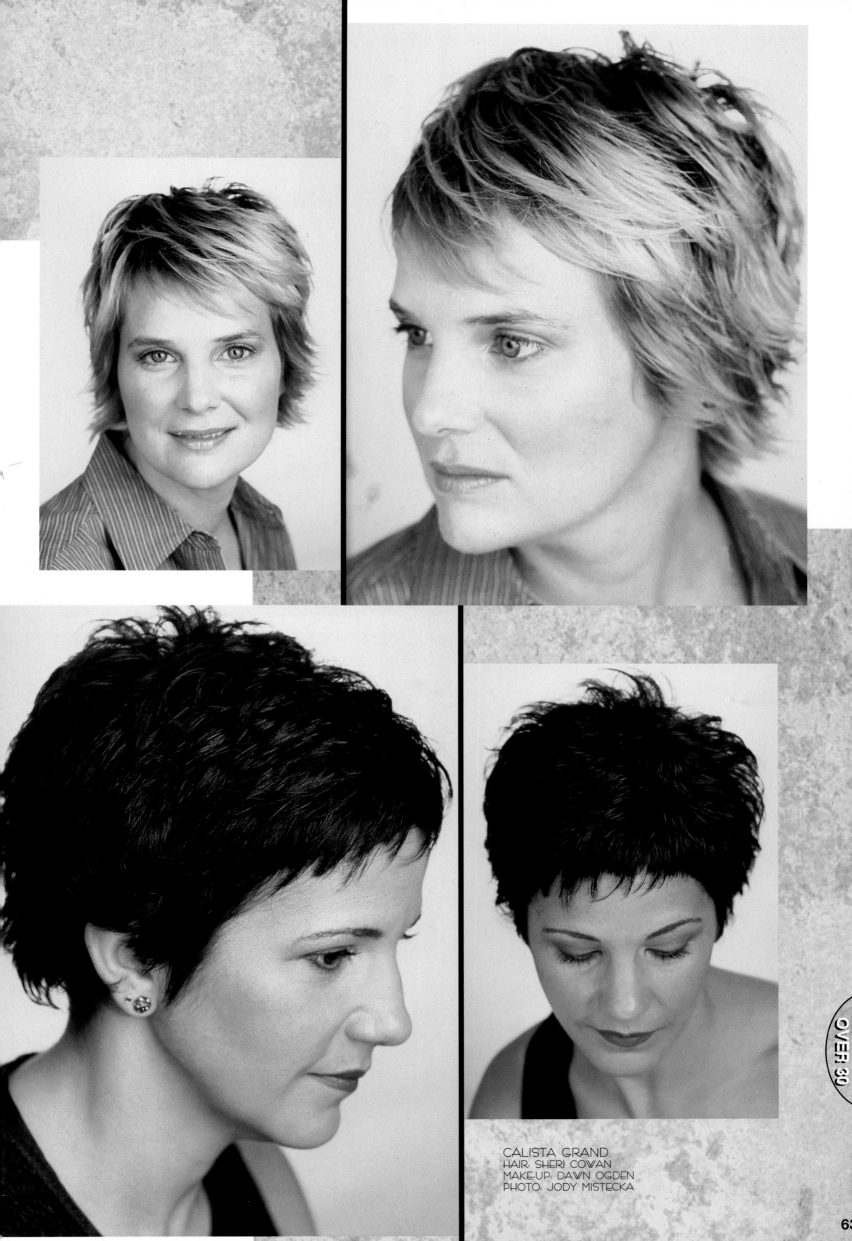

CALISTA GRAND
HAIR: SHERI COWAN
MAKE-UP: DAWN OGDEN
PHOTO: JODY MISTECKA

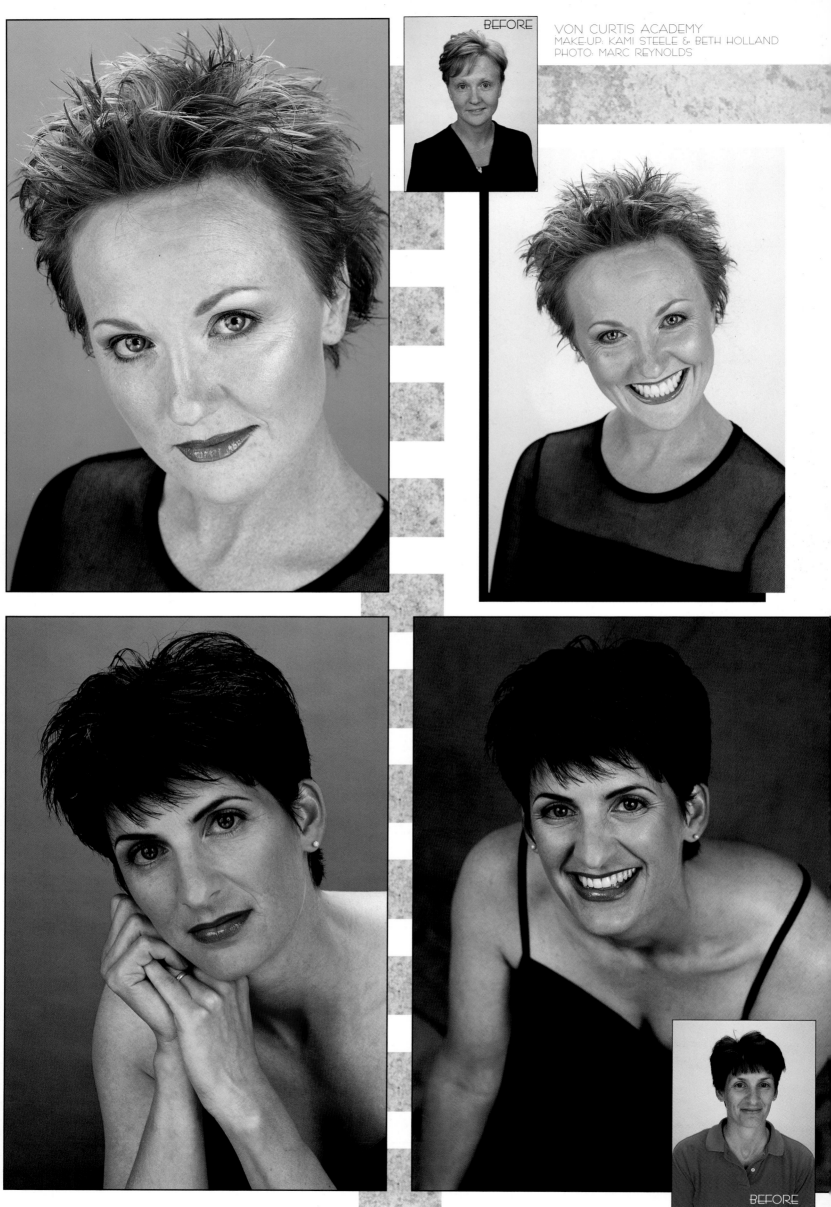

BEFORE

VON CURTIS ACADEMY
MAKE-UP: KAMI STEELE & BETH HOLLAND
PHOTO: MARC REYNOLDS

BEFORE

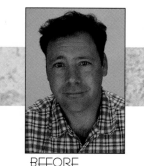

BEFORE

Von Curtis Academy

Model: Eric

Eric is beginning to show the first signs of gray. To create depth we blended and used a semi-permanent color. To enhance his natural wave and update his style, I removed the bulk and razored through extensively.

Tova Stroman

VON CURTIS ACADEMY
MAKE-UP: KAMI STEELE & BETH HOLLAND
PHOTO: MARC REYNOLDS

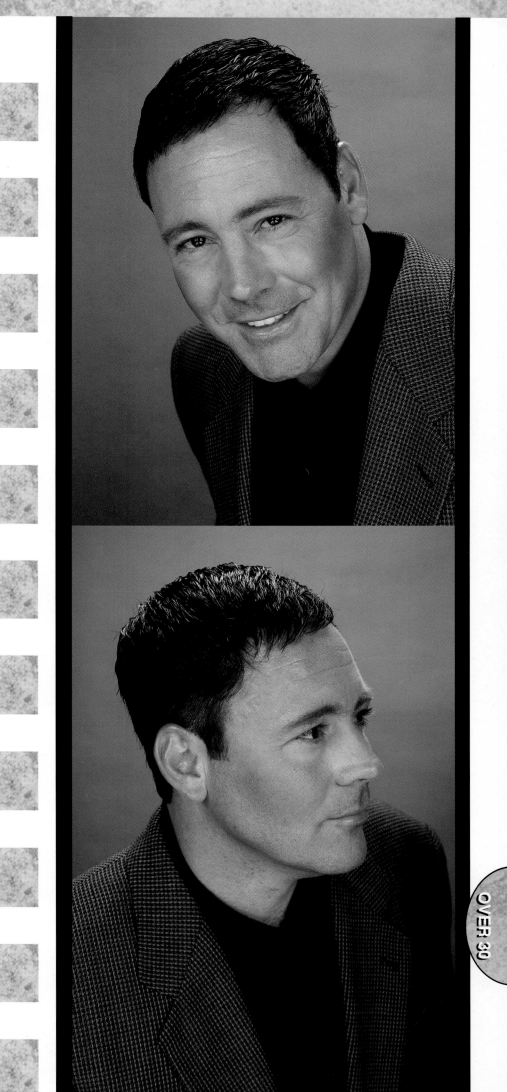

OVER 30

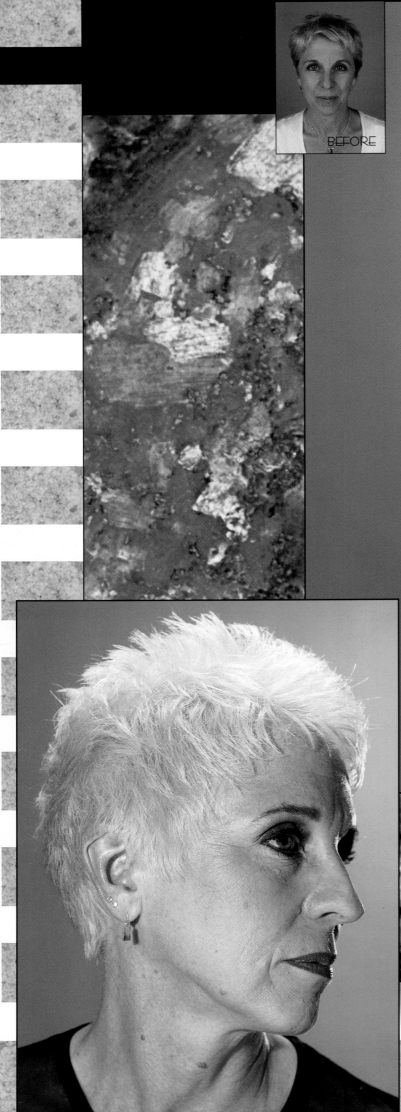

BEFORE

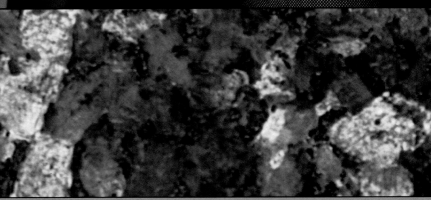

VON CURTIS ACADEMY
MAKE-UP: KAMI STEELE & BETH HOLLAND
PHOTO: MARC REYNOLDS

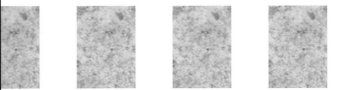

Von Curtis Academy
Model: Donna

Donna needed a new - less age defining look. Something more fun and textured, less matronly. She has naturally red hair that over time has faded quite a bit. I wanted to enhance the red and give her more copper with cinnamon highlights to define the texture we created with the cut.

Dennis James

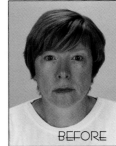

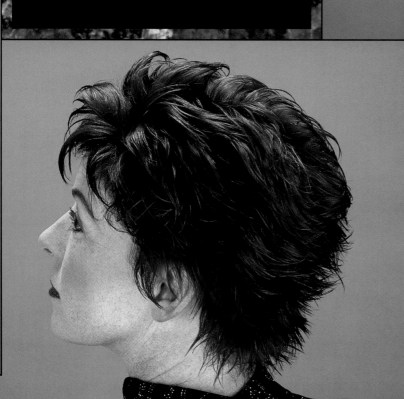

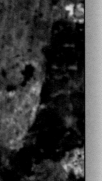

BEFORE

VON CURTIS ACADEMY
MAKE-UP: KAMI STEELE & BETH HOLLAND
PHOTO: MARC REYNOLDS

Von Curtis Academy
Model: Craig

Craig had been growing out his hair and it wasn't working for him. He had been very blond as a child, and gradually his hair darkened. He was in need of a change and we wanted him to look like a GQ model.

Carolyn Nelson

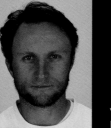

BEFORE

VON CURTIS ACADEMY
MAKE-UP: KAMI STEELE & BETH HOLLAND
PHOTO: MARC REYNOLDS

Von Curtis Academy
Model: Mignonne

Mignonne has naturally curly hair that she normally blows out straight. She was ready for a change, but was afraid to go too short. She has been growing out her fringe - so we decided to blend her lengths to help frame her face. We darkened her natural color and added a few red highlights for a more dramatic look.

Carolyn
Nelson

VON CURTIS ACADEMY
MAKEUP: KAMI STEELE & BETH HOLLAND
PHOTO: MARC REYNOLDS

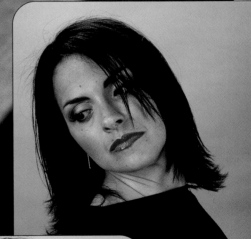

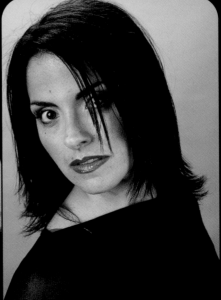

BEFORE

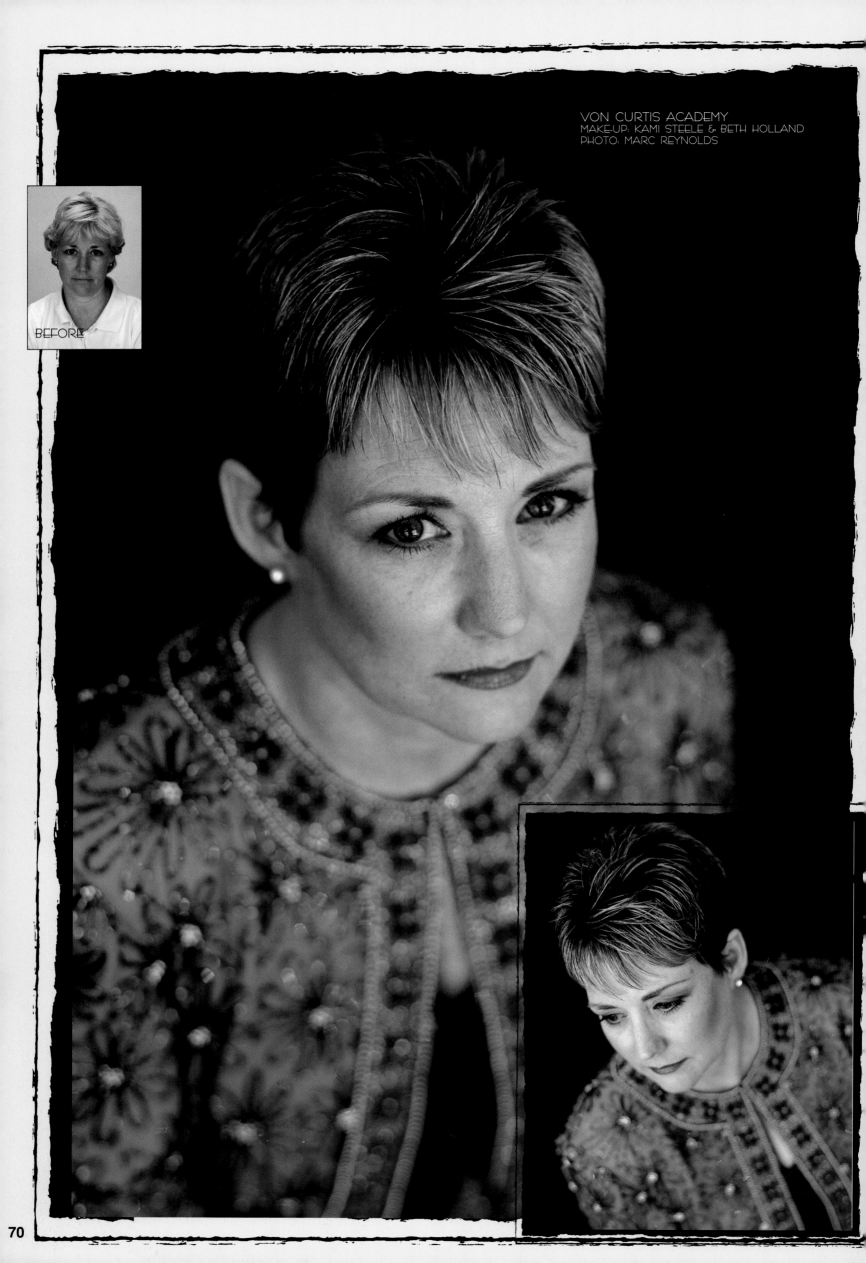

VON CURTIS ACADEMY
MAKE-UP: KAMI STEELE & BETH HOLLAND
PHOTO: MARC REYNOLDS

BEFORE

Von Curtis Academy

Model: Joanne

We decided on this cut to bring out Joanne's almond shaped eyes. The style also helps accentuate her color, and gives her a variety of styling options.
Corinne Jensen

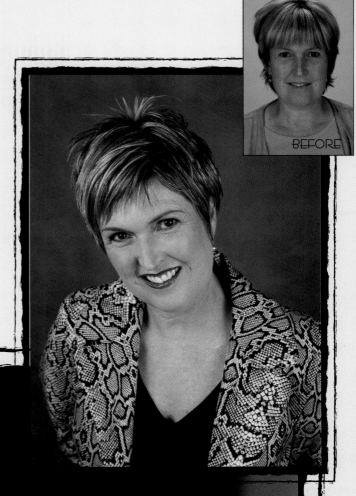

BEFORE

VON CURTIS ACADEMY
MAKE-UP: KAMI STEELE & BETH HOLLAND
PHOTO: MARC REYNOLDS

OVER 30

71

Von Curtis Academy
Model: Alice

I chose this style because Alice's hair is very thick and extremely coarse. She wanted something sassy that suited her lifestyle. This cut is quick and easy for her, and shows off her facial features making her look youthful and sexy.
Cyndi Woodcox

BEFORE

BEFORE

Von Curtis Academy
Model: Leslie

Leslie has been wearing her hair in a variation of a bob for several years. She needed a fun, piecier updated look. This cut offers her the versatility to wear her hair differently with very low maintenance. Her color was quite drab so I added some lighter highlights with some darker blond for contrast.
Carolyn Nelson

VON CURTIS ACADEMY
MAKEUP: KAMI STEELE & BETH HOLLAND
PHOTO: MARC REYNOLDS

Von Curtis Academy

Model: Tim

Tim has been gray since high school. We wanted to change the texture of his hair so we bleached and colored it. His cut is a little more sep- arated to give him multiple styling options.
Mike Helm

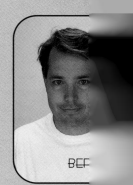

BEF

VON CURTIS ACADEMY
MAKE-UP: KAMI STEELE & BETH HOLLAND
PHOTO: MARC REYNOLDS

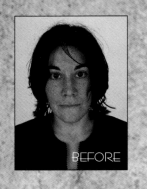

Von Curtis Academy
Model: Lori

Lori had never colored her hair before, and this is why I chose to keep her color subtle. We added a lot of layers and texture to her hair without making it too much shorter. This was a great start for Lori and her new look.
Brennan Claybaugh

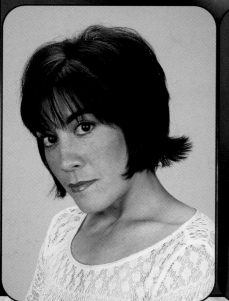

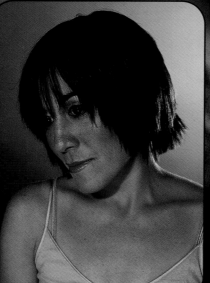

VON CURTIS ACADEMY
MAKE-UP: KAMI STEELE & BETH HOLLAND
PHOTO: MARC REYNOLDS

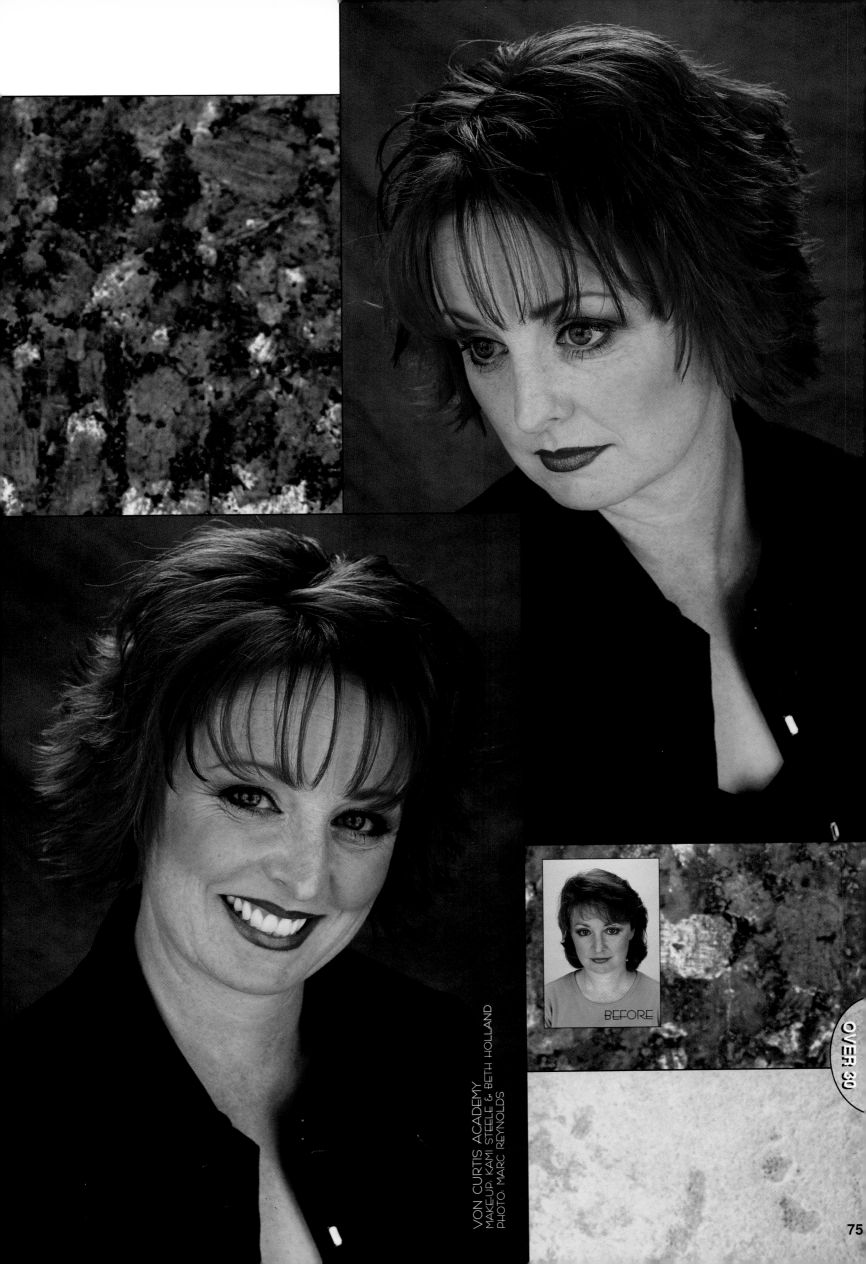

BEFORE

VON CURTIS ACADEMY
MAKEUP: KAMI STEELE & BETH HOLLAND
PHOTO: MARC REYNOLDS

OVER 30

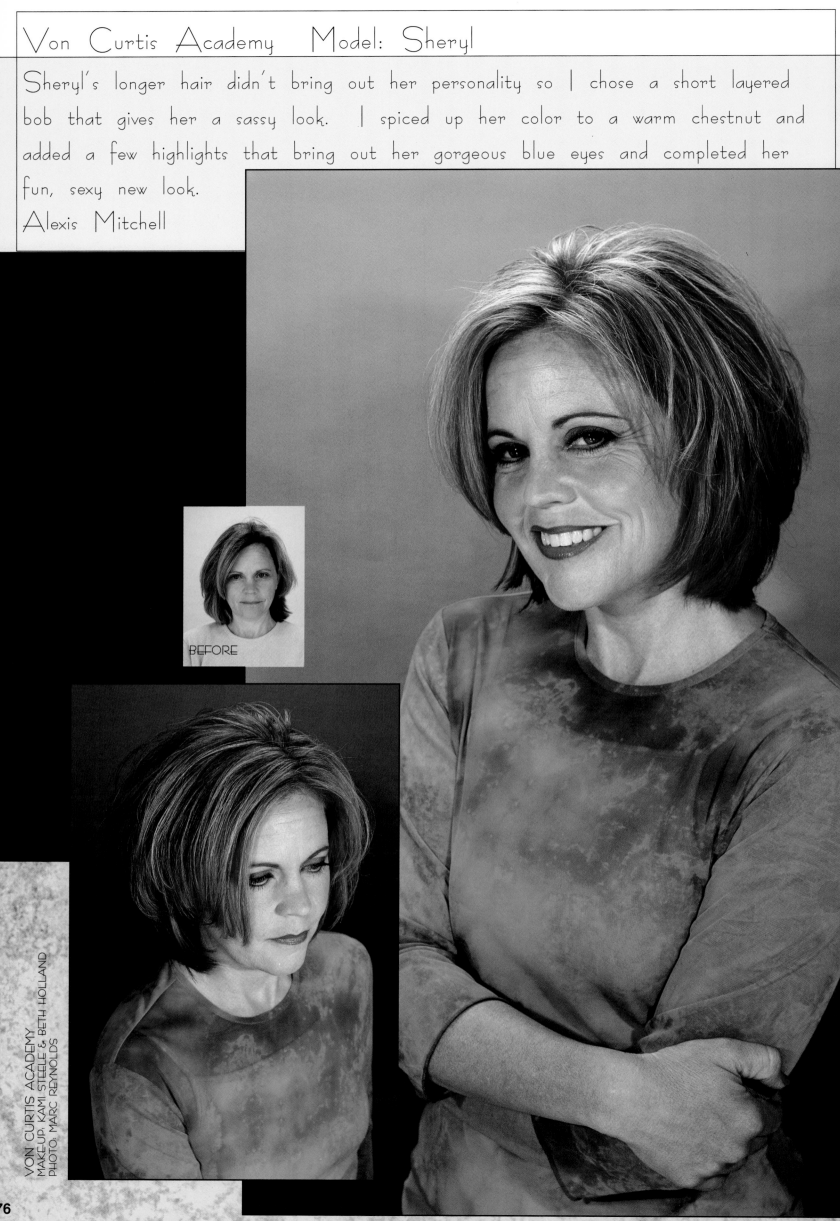

Von Curtis Academy   Model: Sheryl

Sheryl's longer hair didn't bring out her personality so I chose a short layered bob that gives her a sassy look. I spiced up her color to a warm chestnut and added a few highlights that bring out her gorgeous blue eyes and completed her fun, sexy new look.

Alexis Mitchell

BEFORE

VON CURTIS ACADEMY
MAKE-UP: KAMI STEELE & BETH HOLLAND
PHOTO: MARC REYNOLDS

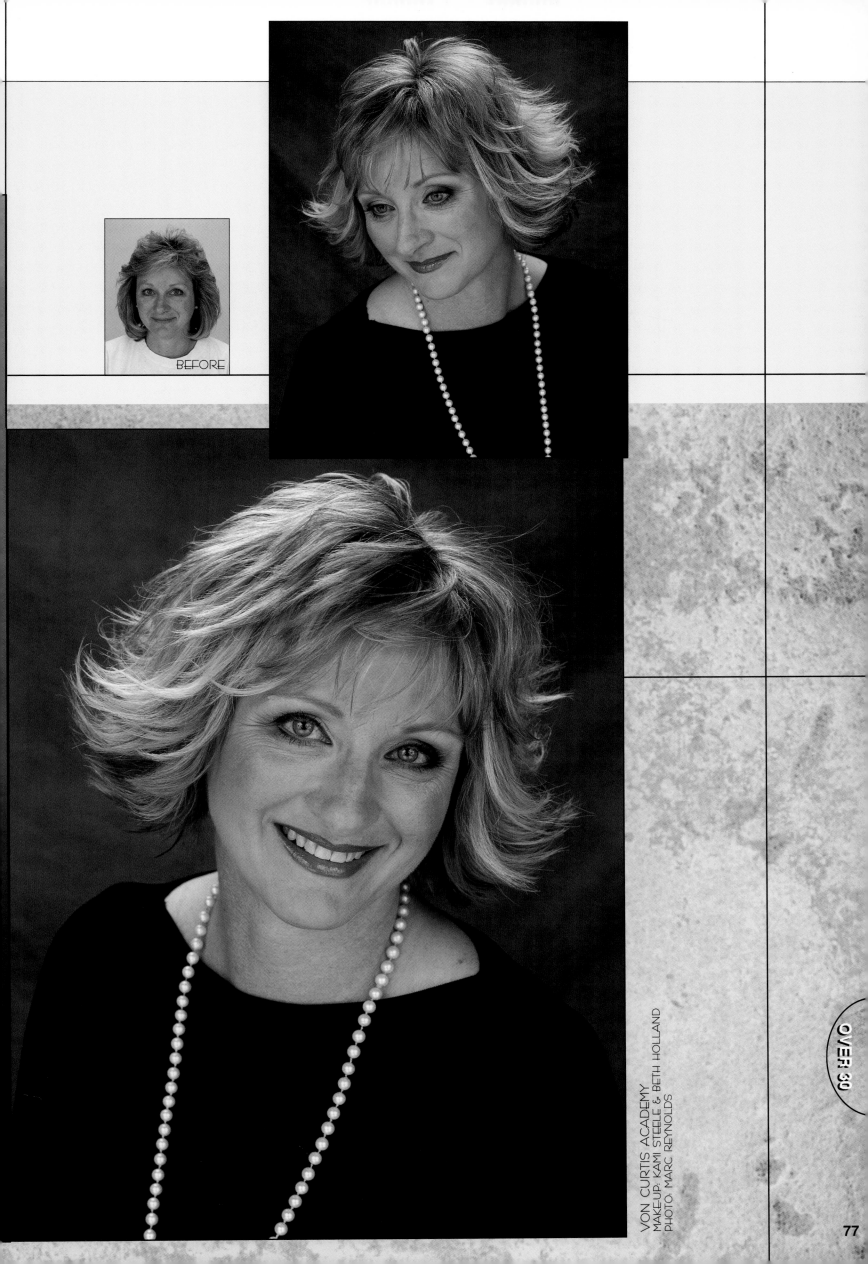

BEFORE

OVER 30

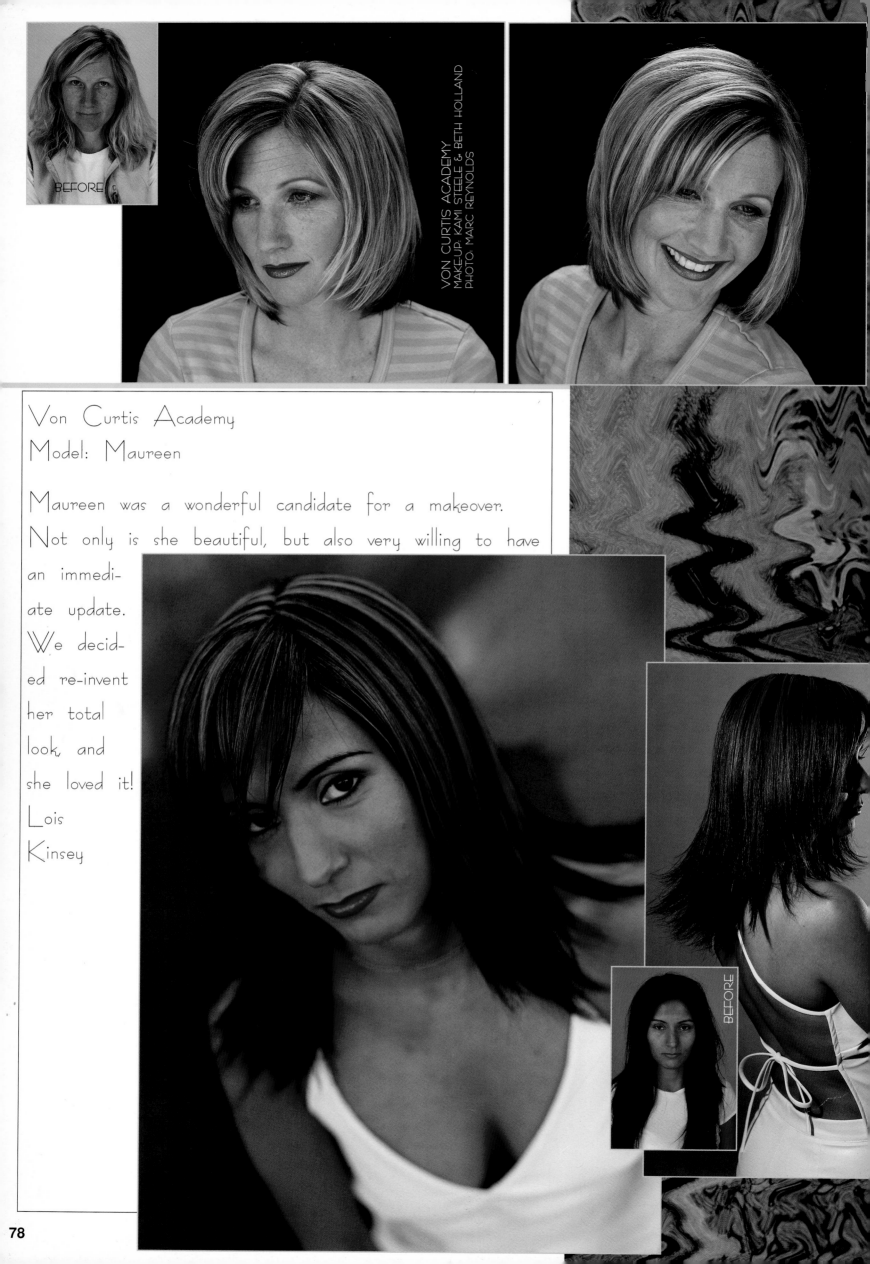

VON CURTIS ACADEMY
MAKEUP: KAMI STEELE & BETH HOLLAND
PHOTO: MARC REYNOLDS

Von Curtis Academy
Model: Maureen

Maureen was a wonderful candidate for a makeover. Not only is she beautiful, but also very willing to have an immediate update. We decided re-invent her total look, and she loved it!
Lois Kinsey

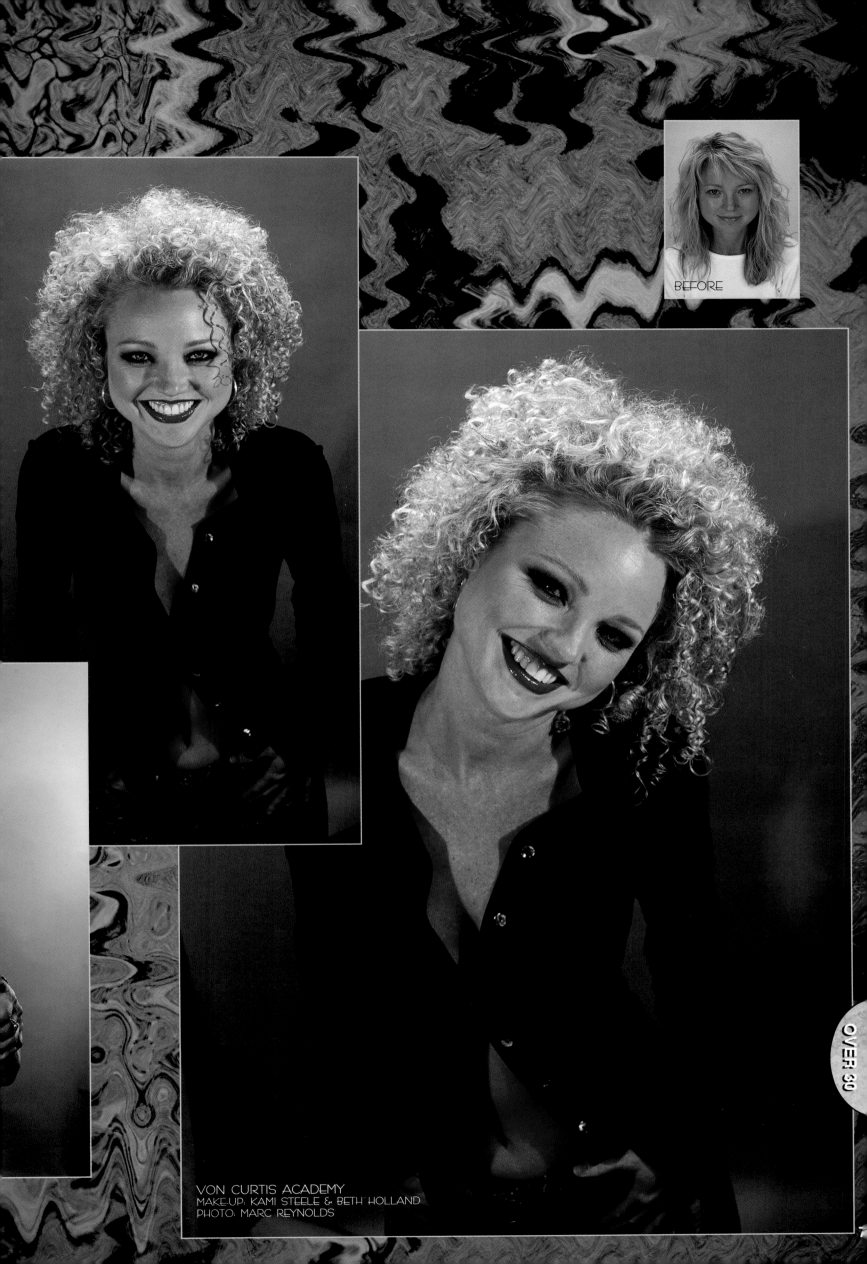

BEFORE

VON CURTIS ACADEMY
MAKE-UP: KAMI STEELE & BETH HOLLAND
PHOTO: MARC REYNOLDS

OVER 30

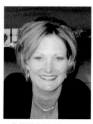

BEFORE

Garbos
Blondes are big this season.
Making a bold statement, Devan loves her new short and spiky look.
Nicole Simmons-Meyers

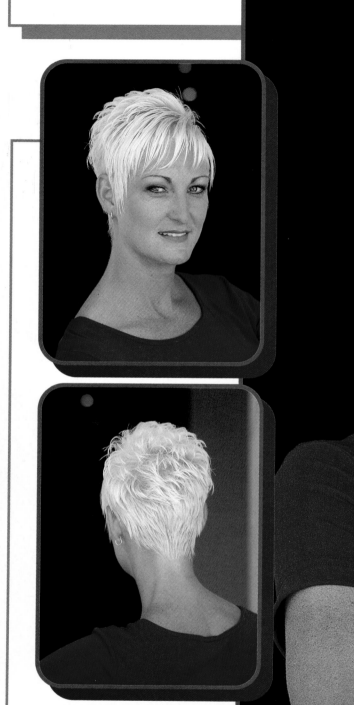

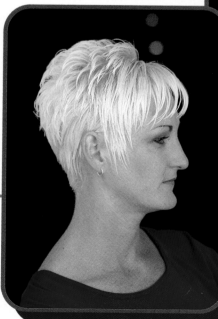

GARBOS
HAIR: NICOLE SIMMONS-MEYERS
MAKE-UP: JAIME QUEENIN
PHOTO: TAGGART-WINTERHALTER

GARBOS
HAIR: NICOLE SIMMONS-MEYERS
MAKE-UP: JAIME QUEENIN
PHOTO: TAGGART-WINTERHALTER

BEFORE

OVER 30

81

Salon Boucle

Laura is a new mom and ease of care is a must. She also wanted something short but professional looking for work. This short wispy style is perfect for her busy lifestyle.

Designer: Stacey Rosenberg

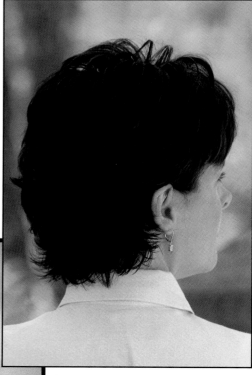

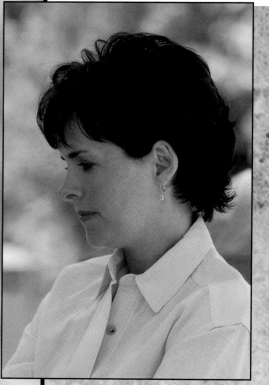

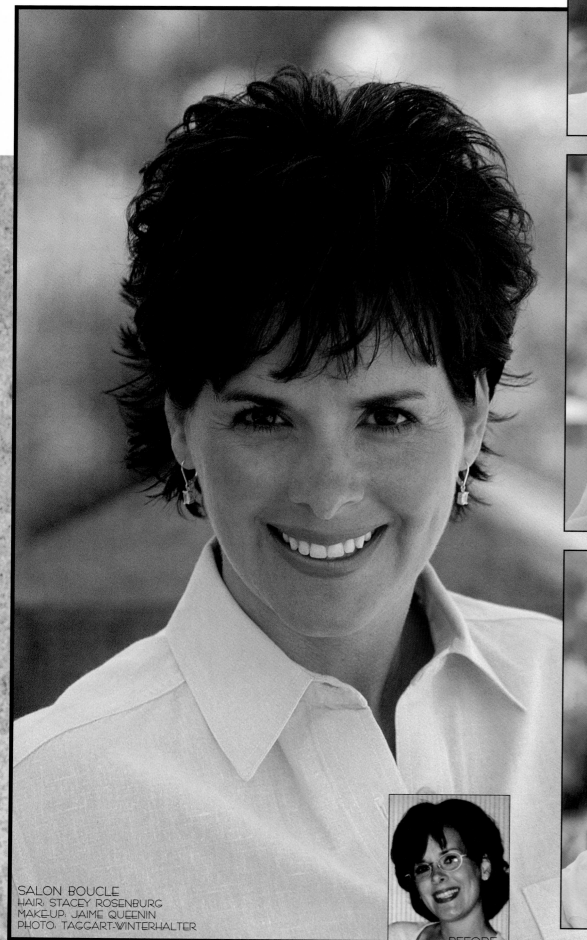

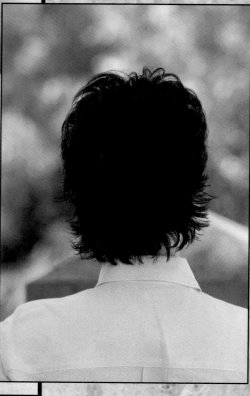

SALON BOUCLE
HAIR: STACEY ROSENBURG
MAKE-UP: JAIME QUEENIN
PHOTO: TAGGART-WINTERHALTER

BEFORE

Salon Boucle

Lisa is a hairdresser herself and is always trying on new looks. She likes to get a little bolder in a shorter length with fun highly dimensional haircolor. Her clients love the new look!

Designer: Katie Rapier

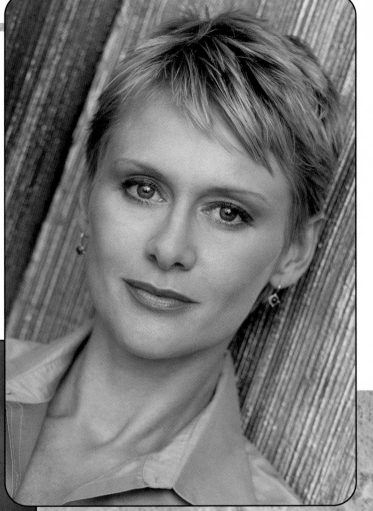

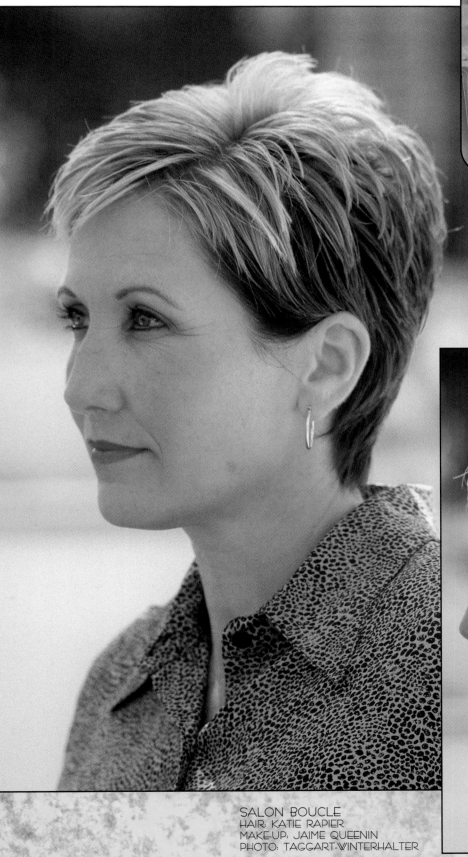

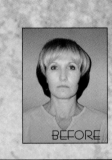

BEFORE

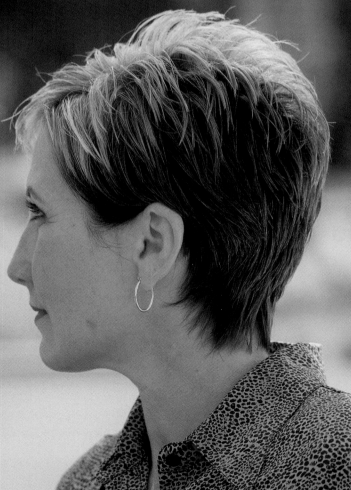

SALON BOUCLE
HAIR: KATIE RAPIER
MAKE-UP: JAIME QUEENIN
PHOTO: TAGGART-WINTERHALTER

OVER 30

Marc and Company

For those like Jennifer who love their length, texture and haircolor have many options for a new look. After straightening, thinly sliced highlights were added for warmth and dimension. A gloss over the top seals in the color and gives a glassy finish.

Designer:
Ping
Latvong

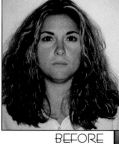
BEFORE

MARC AND COMPANY
HAIR: PING LATVONG
MAKE-UP: JAIME QUEENIN

Centerstage Salon and Day Spa

Patti has had a perm for years and wanted something more sleek and manageable. She also wanted to go blonde versus strawberry for color.

Designer:
Monica
Salena
Martinez

BEFORE

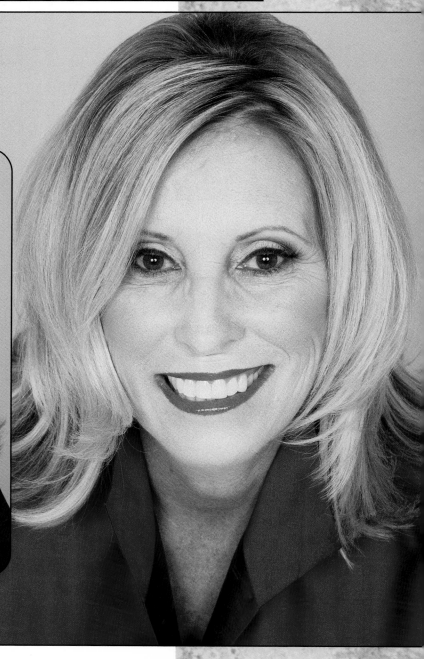

CENTERSTAGE SALON AND DAY SPA
HAIR: MONICA SALENA MARTINEZ   MAKE-UP: MONICA SALENA MARTINEZ
PHOTO: TAGGART-WINTERHALTER

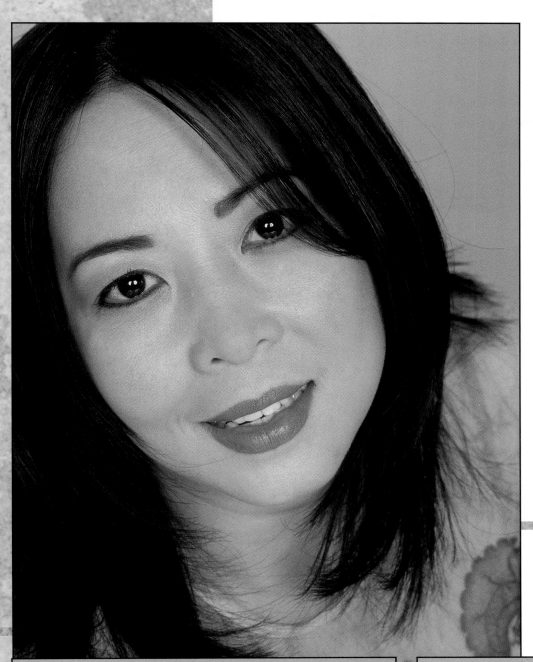

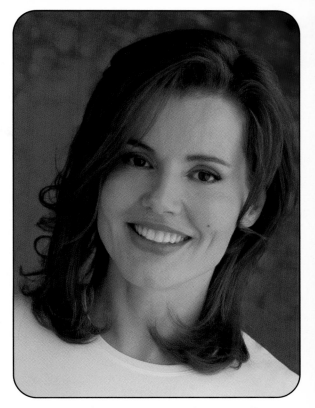

Style Influenced by Geena Davis

Salon Boucle

Sometimes a simple change can give very dramatic results.

Designer Jolene Torres

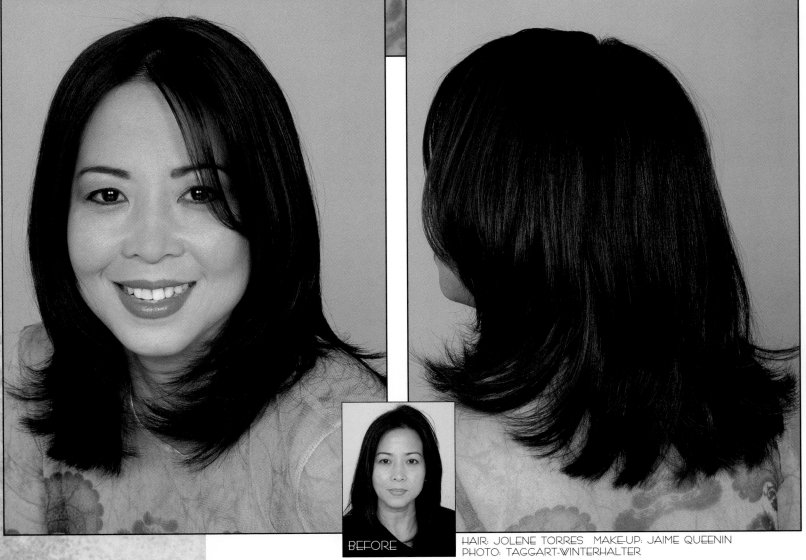

BEFORE

HAIR: JOLENE TORRES MAKE-UP: JAIME QUEENIN
PHOTO: TAGGART-WINTERHALTER

Victor Paul

Both Stacie and Jane like a hip and young look. These are two different length versions of an updated flip that have a definite 70's flair. Instead of a flip upward only toward the bottom, these kick outward and away from the face.

Victor Paul

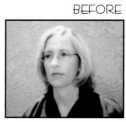

VICTOR PAUL
MAKEUP: JAIME QUEENIN
PHOTO: TAGGART-WINTERHALTER

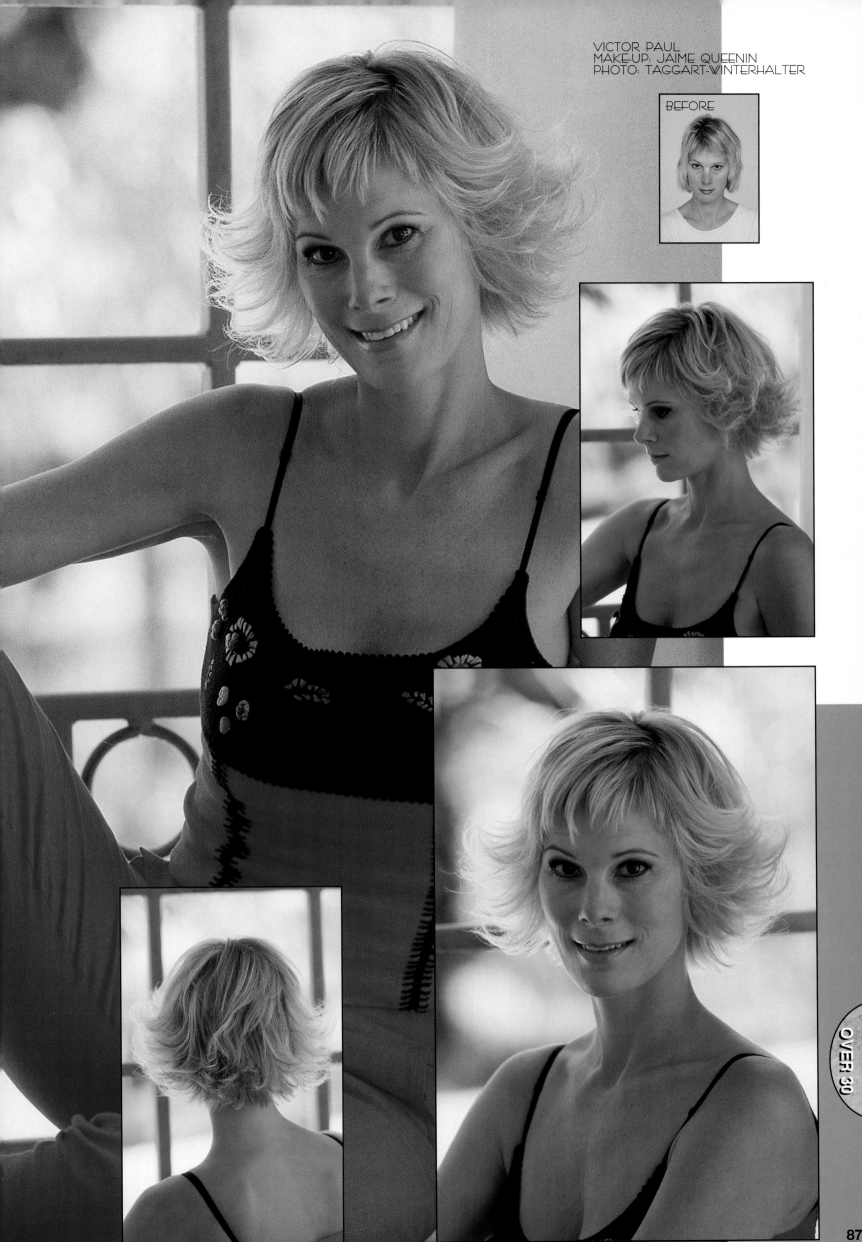

VICTOR PAUL
MAKE-UP: JAIME QUEENIN
PHOTO: TAGGART-WINTERHALTER

BEFORE

OVER 30

87

Salon Boucle

A perfect style update, Sherrie wanted a change without going too drastic. A rounded mid length style frames her face nicely, while a rich coppery red color scream for attention.

Designer: Mehran

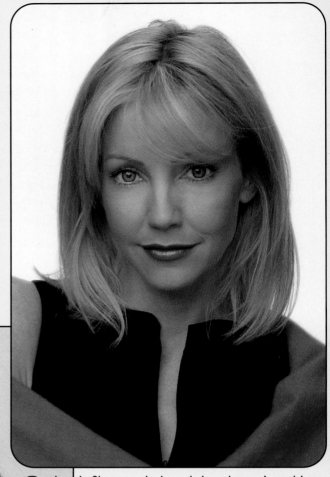

Style Influenced by Heather Locklear

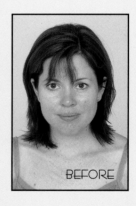

BEFORE

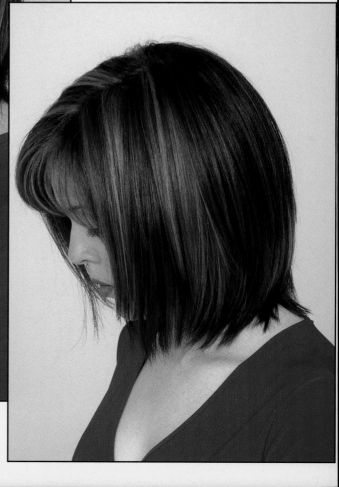

SALON BOUCLE
HAIR: MEHRAN
MAKE-UP: JAIME QUEENIN
PHOTO: TAGGART-WINTERHALTER

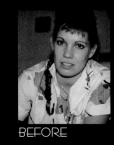

Salon De'Dawn

Sheila likes to walk on the wild side. With her new lighter, shorter look, she's finding that blondes definitely do have more fun!

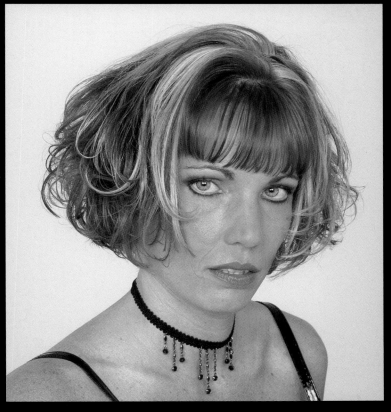

SALON DE'DAWN
HAIR: DAWN ORLOW-TOWNSEND   MAKE-UP: JAIME QUEENIN
PHOTO: TAGGART-WINTERHALTER

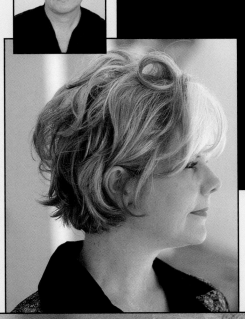

Salon Boucle

Annemarie has a sophisticated piecey look that can be worn casual with jeans, or dressed up for evening and business.

Designer: Jamie McIntyre

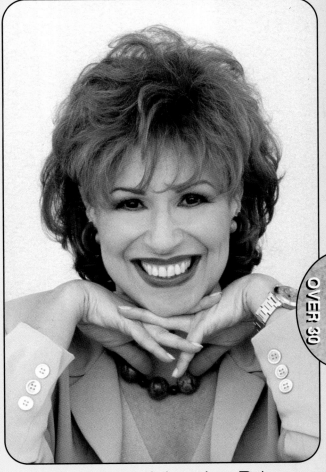

SALON DE'DAWN
HAIR: JAMIE MCINTYRE
MAKE-UP: JAIME QUEENIN
PHOTO: TAGGART-WINTERHALTER

Style Influenced by Joy Behar

OVER 30

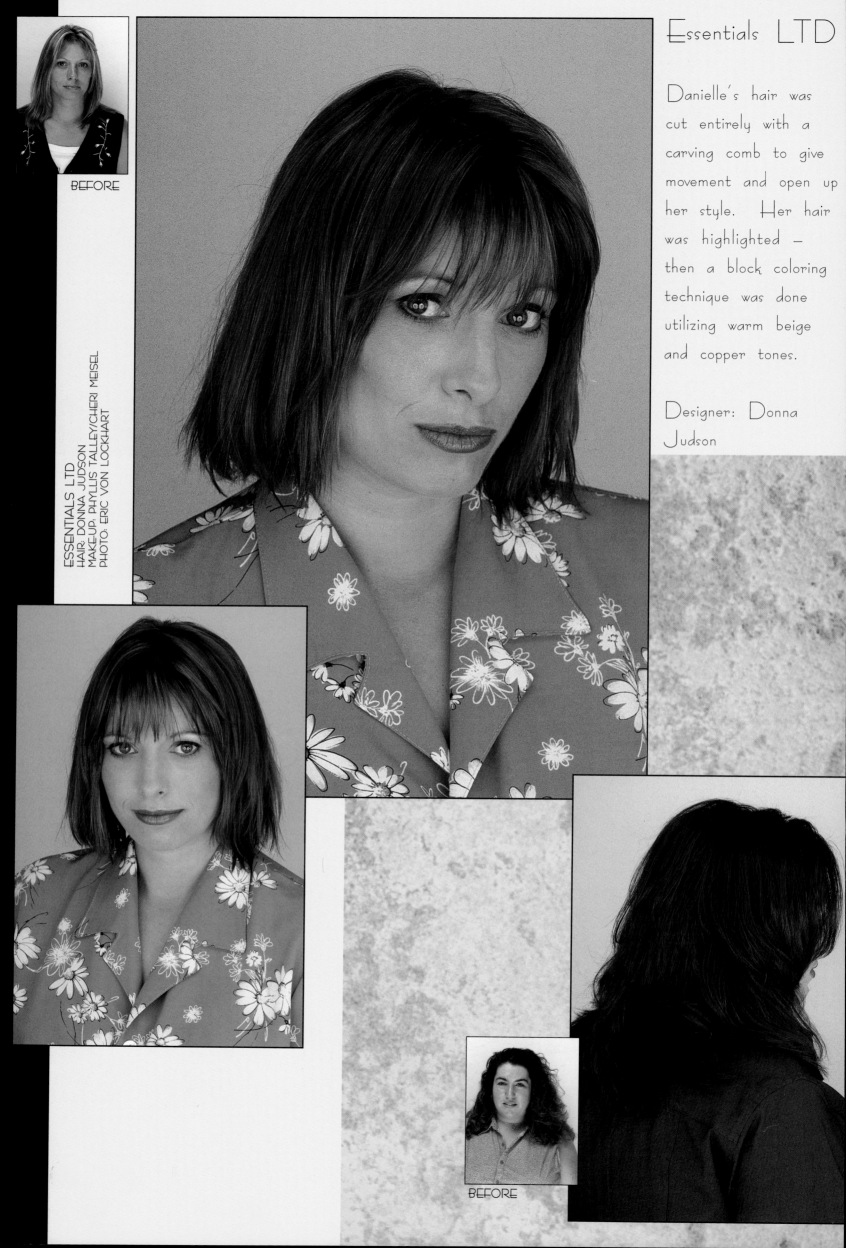

Danielle's hair was cut entirely with a carving comb to give movement and open up her style. Her hair was highlighted — then a block coloring technique was done utilizing warm beige and copper tones.

Designer: Donna Judson

ESSENTIALS LTD
HAIR: DONNA JUDSON
MAKE-UP: PHYLLIS TALLEY/CHERI MEISEL
PHOTO: ERIC VON LOCKHART

BEFORE

BEFORE

90

ESSENTIALS LTD
HAIR: PERLE NORMANDIN
MAKE-UP: PHYLLIS TALLEY/CHERI MEISEL
PHOTO: ERIC VON LOCKHART

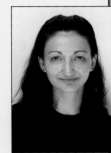

BEFORE

Amy's natural curly hair was cut just below the shoulders with low graduations to remove excess bulk. To draw attention to her eyes and cheekbones sections were sliced out using ARC scissors.

Dimension and shine were added with rich red color.

OVER 30

ESSENTIALS LTD
HAIR: DONNA JUDSON
MAKE-UP: PHYLLIS TALLEY/CHERI MEISEL
PHOTO: ERIC VON LOCKHART

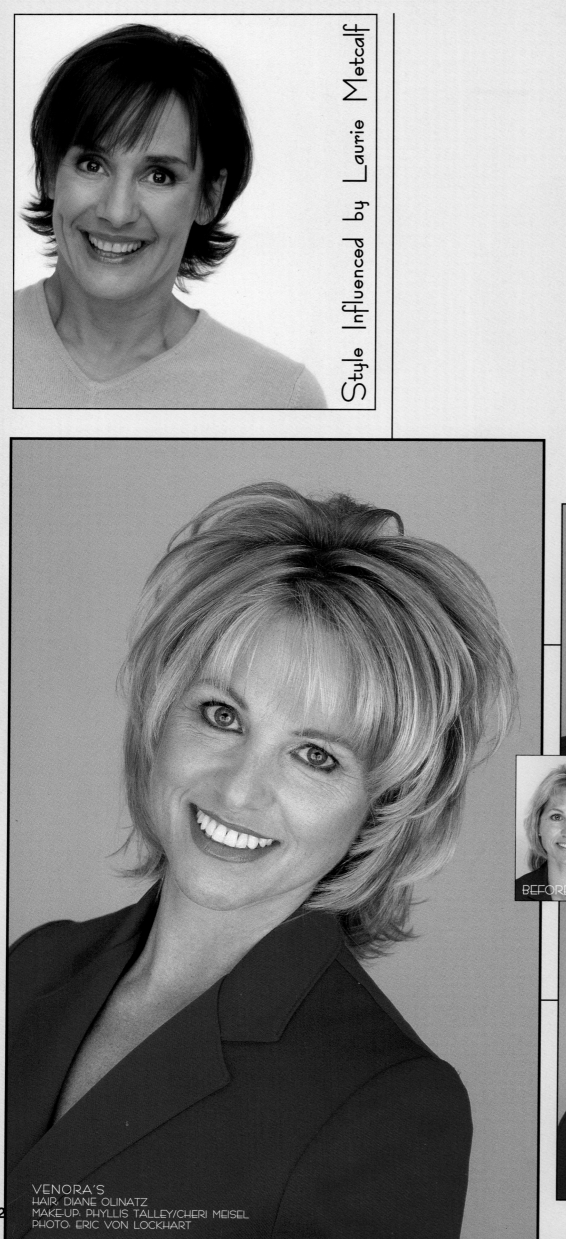

Style Influenced by Laurie Metcalf

VENORA'S
HAIR: KELLY VAIL
MAKE-UP: PHYLLIS TALLEY/CHERI MEISEL
PHOTO: ERIC VON LOCKHART

BEFORE

VENORA'S
HAIR: DIANE OLINATZ
MAKE-UP: PHYLLIS TALLEY/CHERI MEISEL
PHOTO: ERIC VON LOCKHART

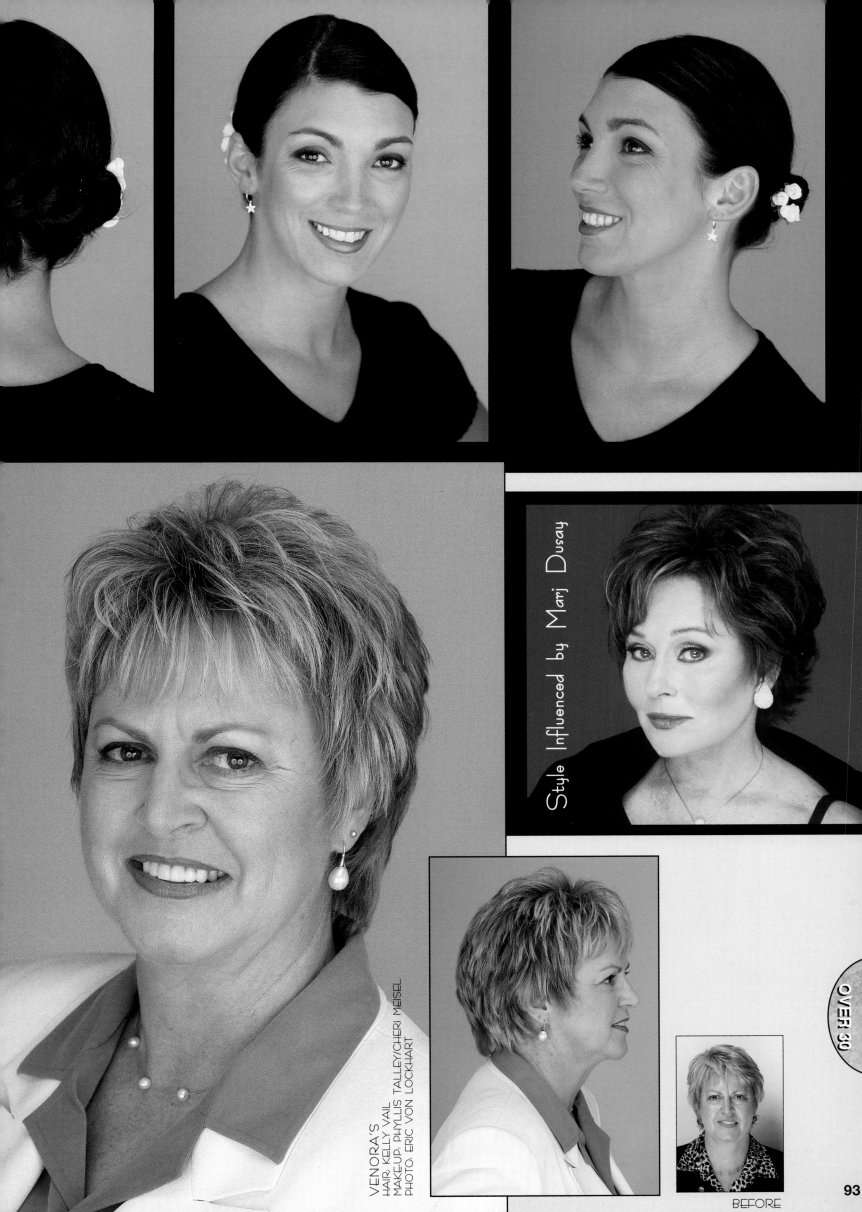

Style Influenced by Marj Dusay

VENORA'S
HAIR: KELLY VAIL
MAKE-UP: PHYLLIS TALLEY/CHERI MEISEL
PHOTO: ERIC VON LOCKHART

OVER 30

BEFORE

93

Livolsi

Bob needed a business look. He has thick, curly, unruly hair that is premature gray. I colored his hair to blend the gray using a color two shades lighter than his natural color. I kept the cut close on the sides and back, then used gel and finger raked the top for a more controlled look. To finish off I shaped his eyebrows for a more professional look.

Designer: Christine Livolsi

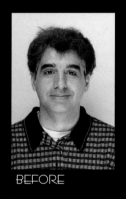

BEFORE

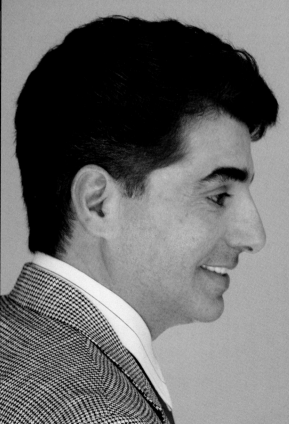

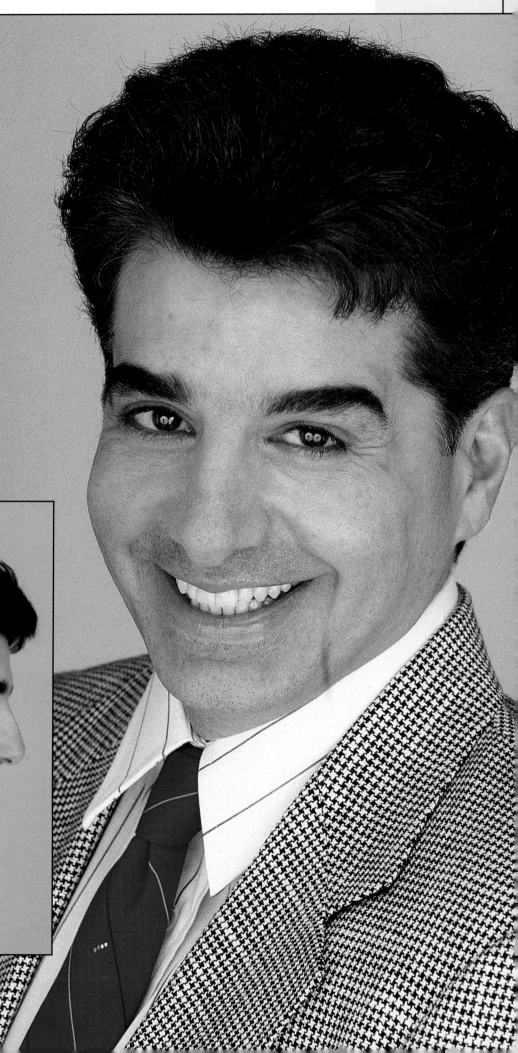

LIVOLSI
HAIR: CHRISTINE LIVOLSI
MAKE-UP: PHYLLIS TALLEY/CHERI MEISEL
PHOTO: ERIC VON LOCKHART

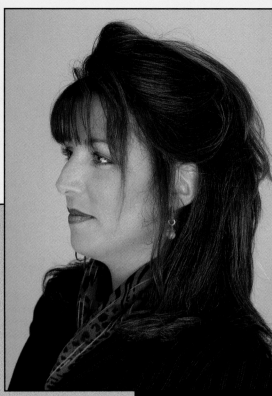

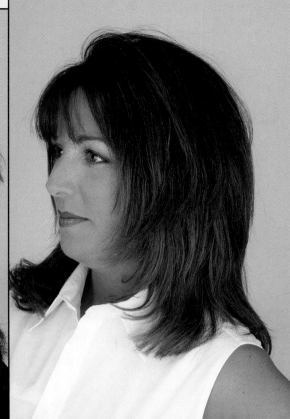

Livolsi

Renee is a ballet dancer who also needs a business look. She needed a versatile cut that could go up or down. The length was kept and shorter pieces were added to frame her face. A rich brown was added for highlight and shine.

Designer: Tine Crocco

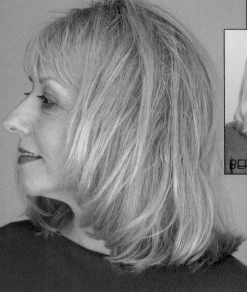

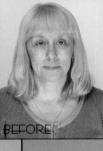

BEFORE

Livolsi

Roberta has thin hair that needed lifting and volume though she did not want to go short. Long layers were cut to frame the face and add fullness. Bangs were added for balance, as well as highlights for a dimensional look. This style can be worn up or down.

OVER 30

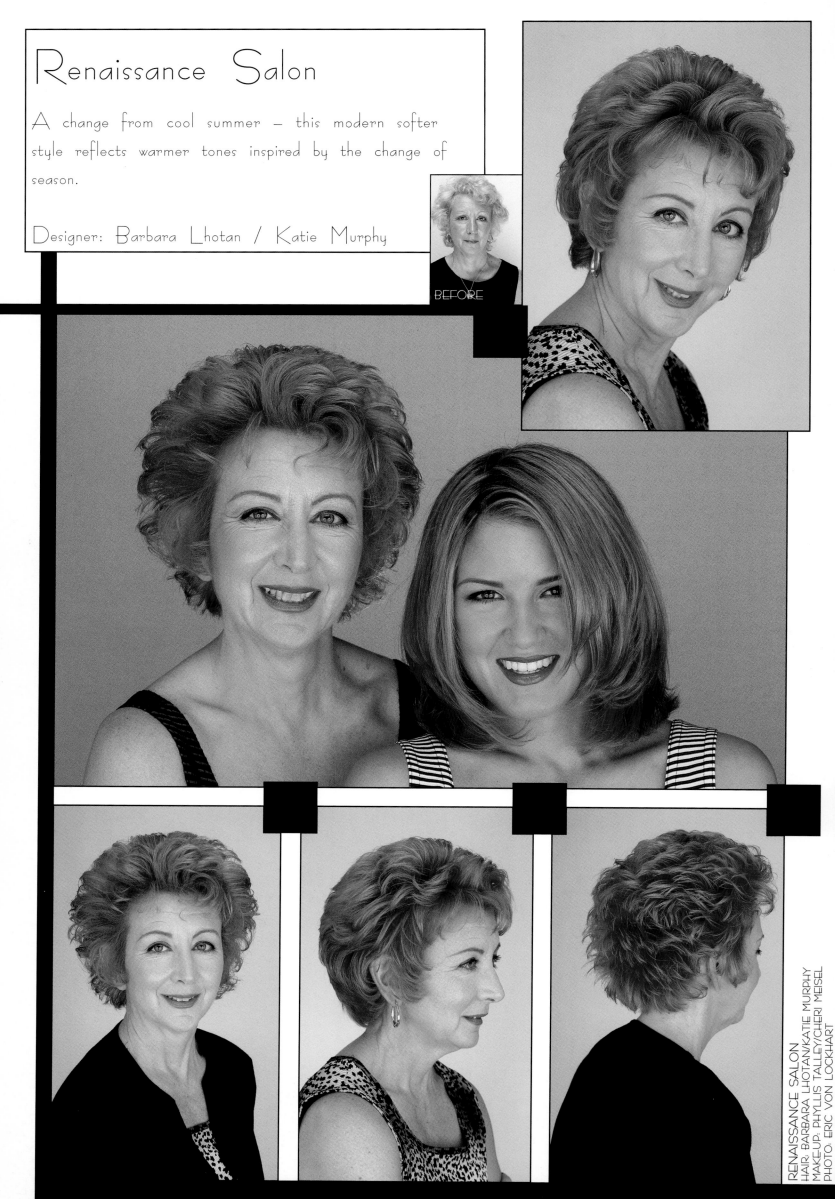

Renaissance Salon

A change from cool summer — this modern softer style reflects warmer tones inspired by the change of season.

Designer: Barbara Lhotan / Katie Murphy

BEFORE

RENAISSANCE SALON
HAIR: BARBARA LHOTAN/KATIE MURPHY
MAKE-UP: PHYLLIS TALLEY/CHERI MEISEL
PHOTO: ERIC VON LOCKHART

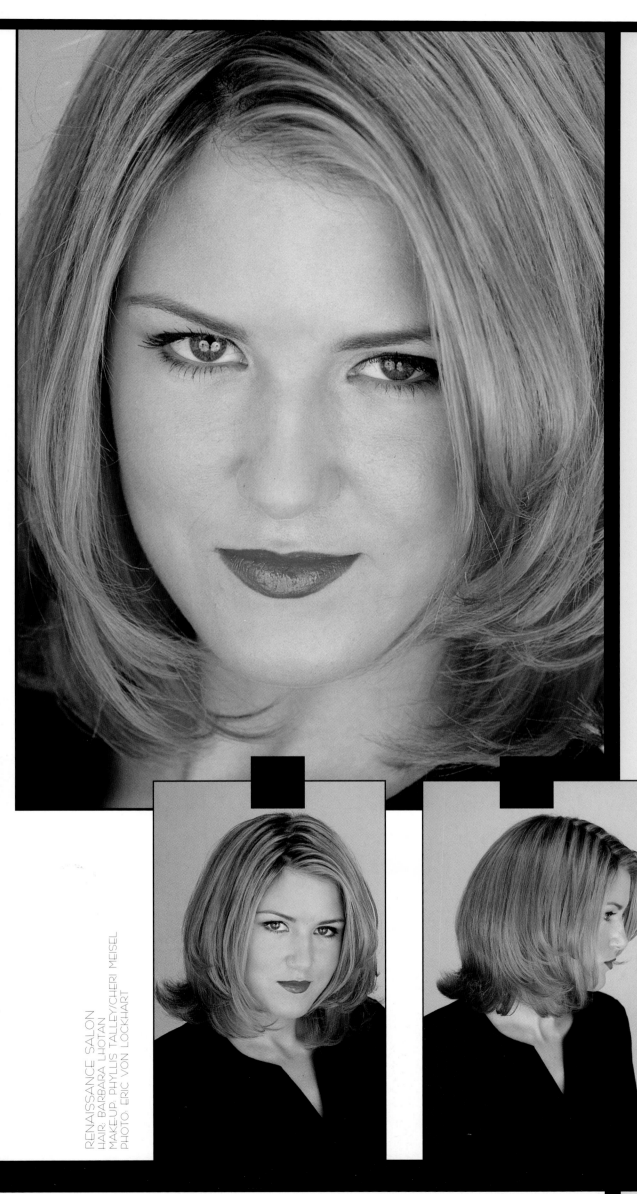

Renaissance Salon

Cotton candy coated for a fun summer look.

Designer:
Barbara Lhotan

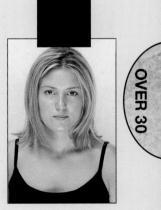

BEFORE

RENAISSANCE SALON
HAIR: BARBARA LHOTAN
MAKEUP: PHYLLIS TALLEY/CHERI MEISEL
PHOTO: ERIC VON LOCKHART

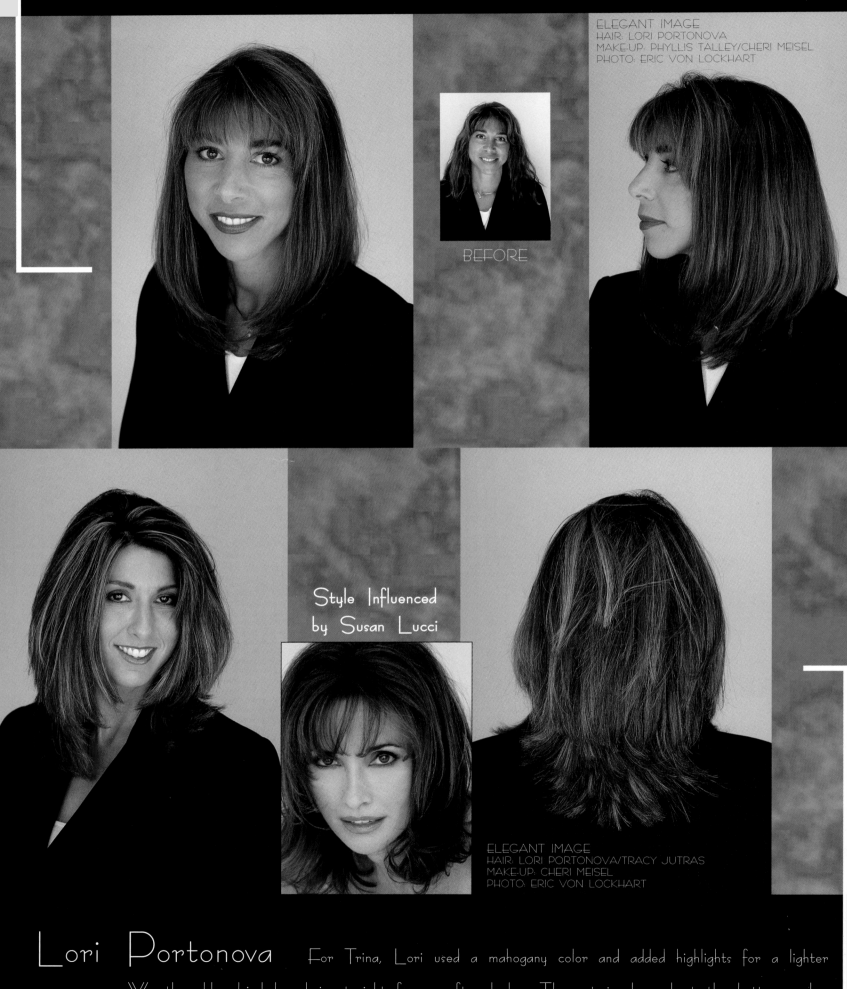

and sophisticated look. Highlights were added to soften her facial features giving a more youthful look.
Designer: Lori Portonova

ELEGANT IMAGE
HAIR: LORI PORTONOVA
MAKE-UP: PHYLLIS TALLEY/CHERI MEISEL
PHOTO: ERIC VON LOCKHART

BEFORE

Style Influenced
by Susan Lucci

ELEGANT IMAGE
HAIR: LORI PORTONOVA/TRACY JUTRAS
MAKE-UP: CHERI MEISEL
PHOTO: ERIC VON LOCKHART

Lori Portonova   For Trina, Lori used a mahogany color and added highlights for a lighter

appearance. We then blow-dried her hair straight for a softer look. The cut is shagged at the bottom and

the length is long on top for fullness   Designer: Lori Portonova / Tracy Jutras

Elegant image

With Rose, we chose a more contemporary bob that is slightly shorter in the nape and slightly longer in the front.   This style gives her a conservative yet trendy look.

Designer: Lori Portonova

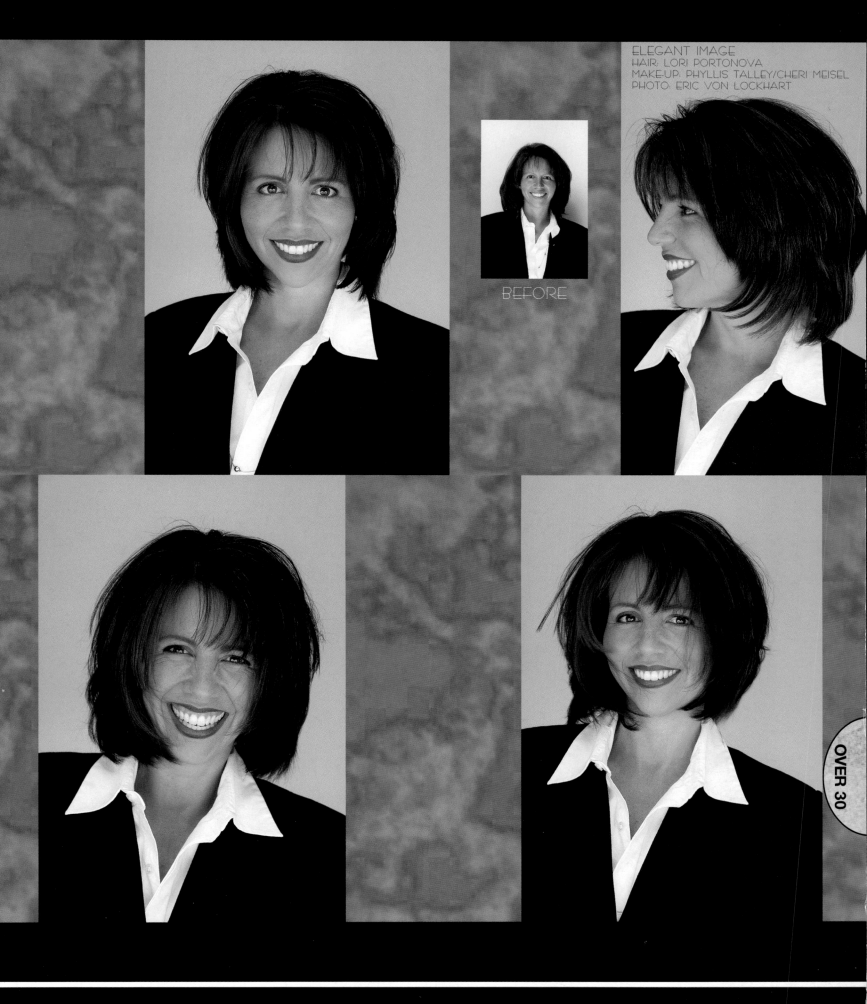

ELEGANT IMAGE
HAIR: LORI PORTONOVA
MAKE-UP: PHYLLIS TALLEY/CHERI MEISEL
PHOTO: ERIC VON LOCKHART

BEFORE

OVER 30

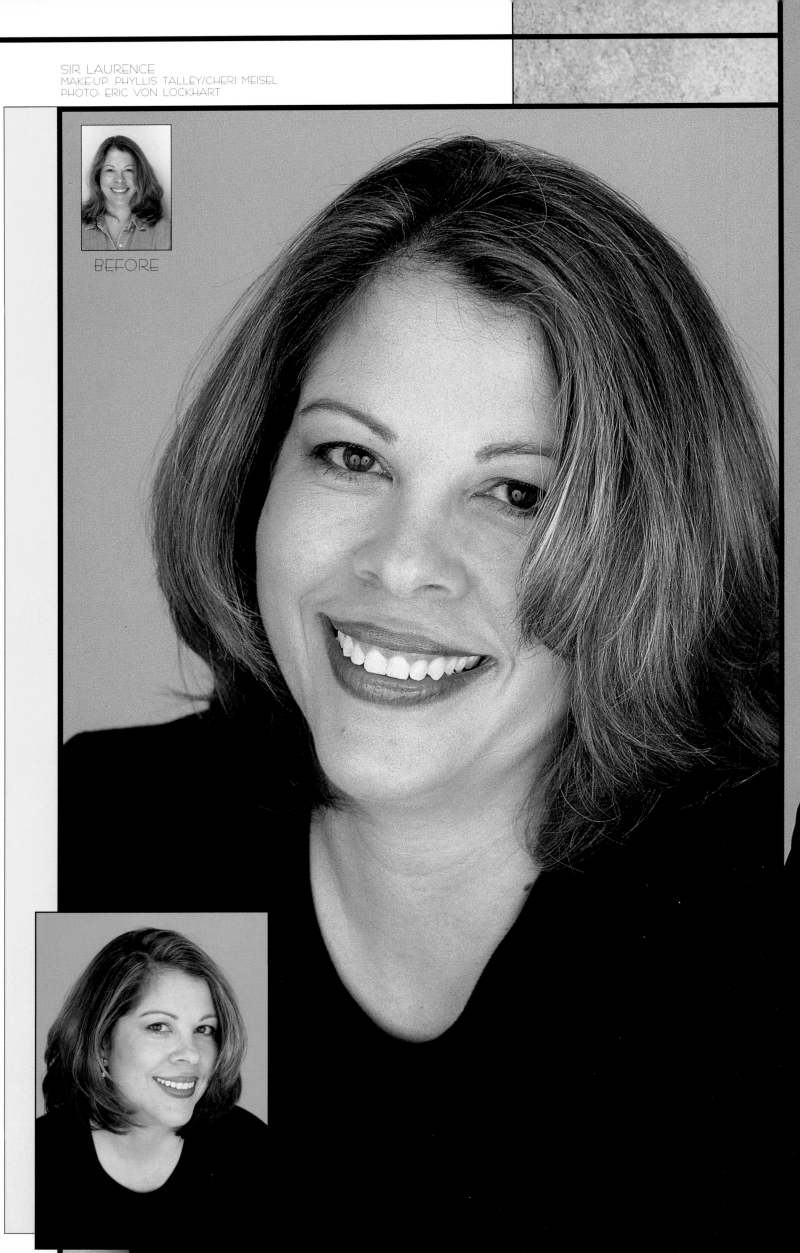

SIR LAURENCE
MAKE-UP: PHYLLIS TALLEY/CHERI MEISEL
PHOTO: ERIC VON LOCKHART

BEFORE

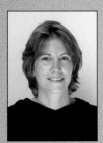

BEFORE

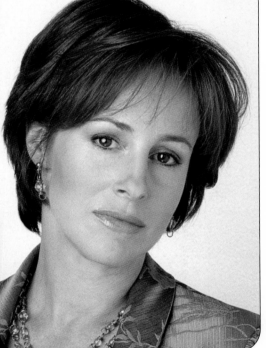

Style Influenced by
Hillary B. Smith

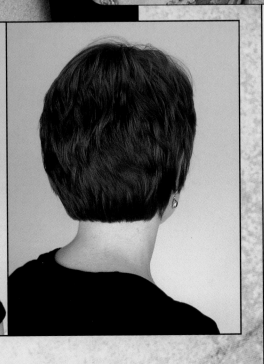

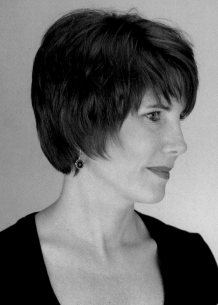

SIR LAURENCE
MAKEUP: PHYLLIS TALLEY/CHERI MEISEL
PHOTO: ERIC VON LOCKHART

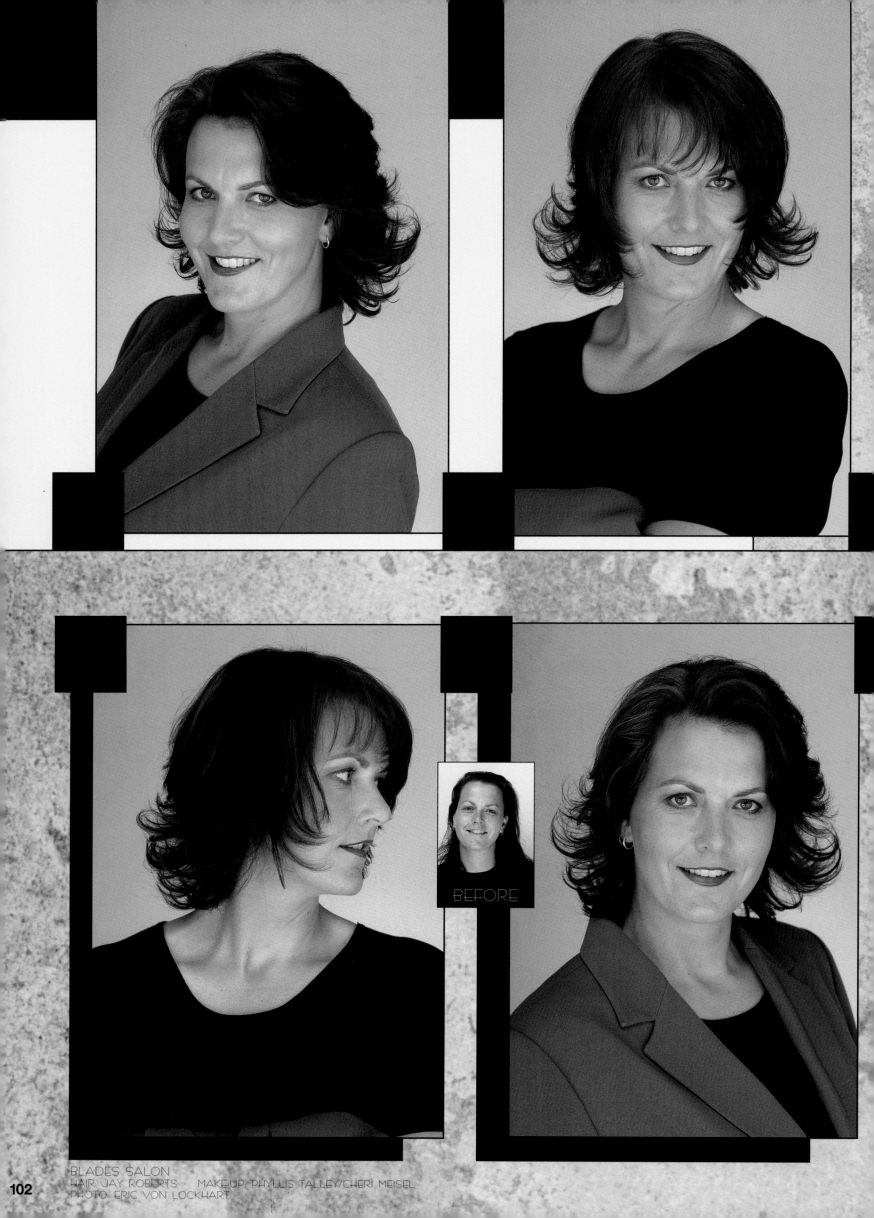

BEFORE

BLADES SALON
HAIR: JAY ROBERTS   MAKE-UP: PHYLLIS TALLEY/CHERI MEISEL
PHOTO: ERIC VON LOCKHART

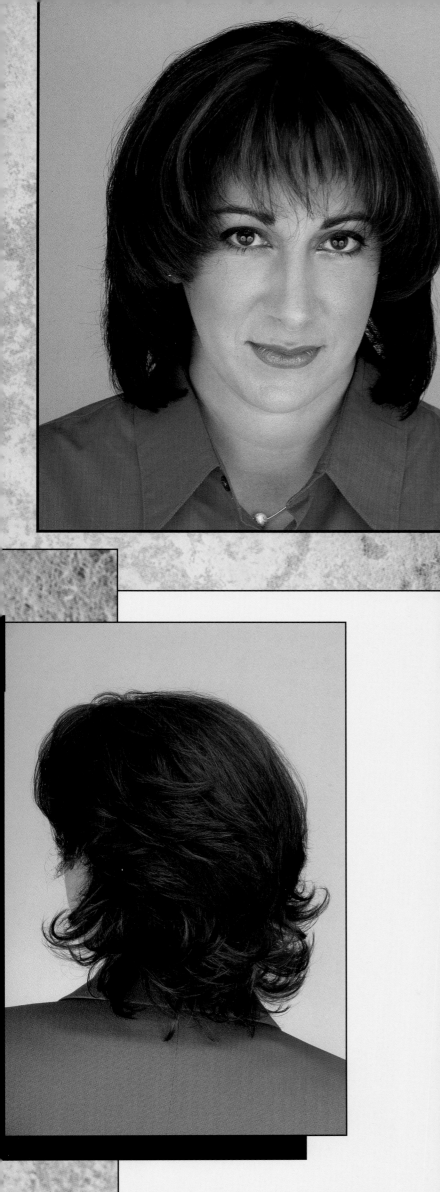

LOOKING GOOD
HAIR: PATTY BACKES
MAKE-UP: PHYLLIS TALLEY/CHERI MEISEL
PHOTO: ERIC VON LOCKHART

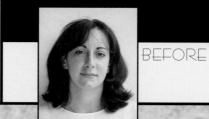

BEFORE

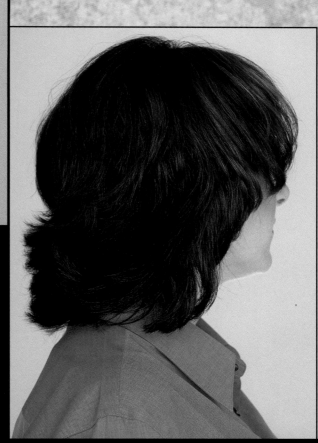

OVER 30

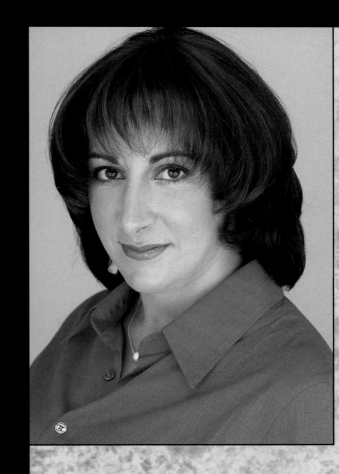

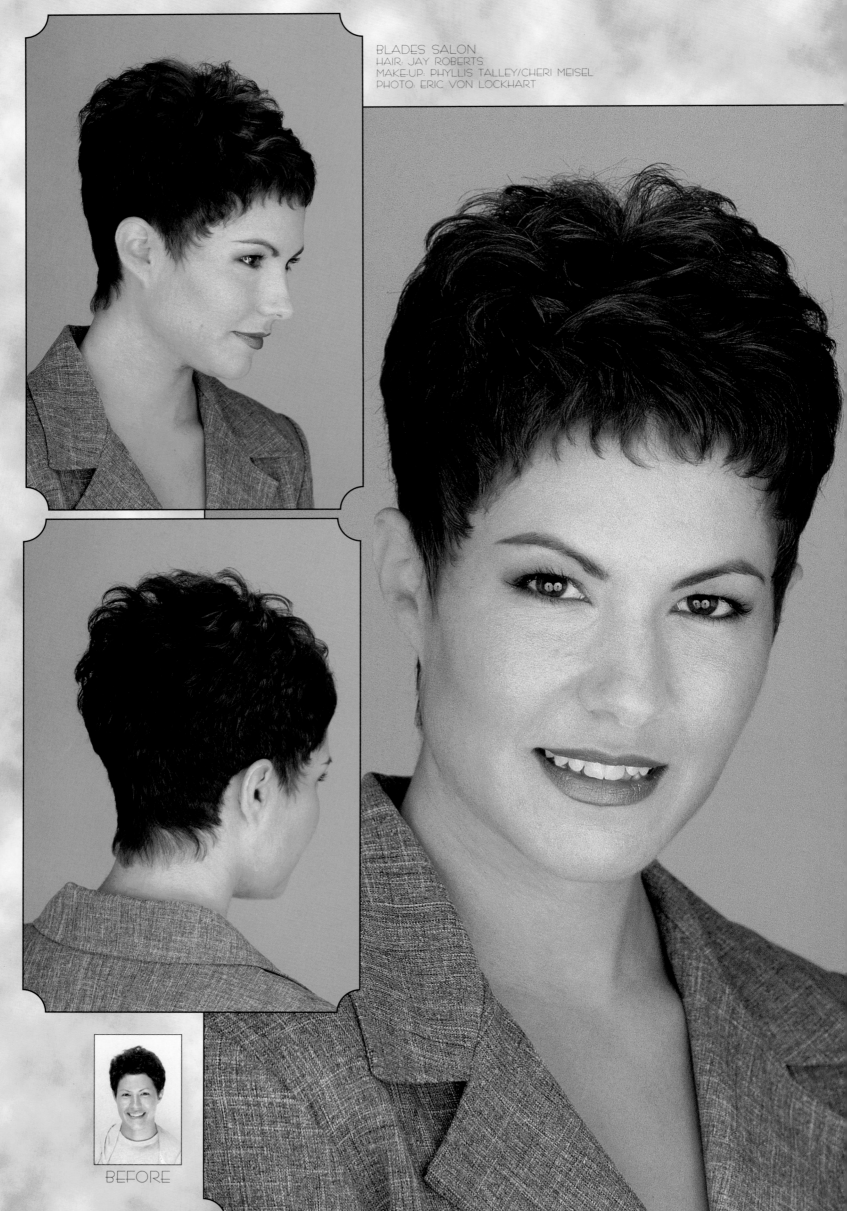

BLADES SALON
HAIR: JAY ROBERTS
MAKE-UP: PHYLLIS TALLEY/CHERI MEISEL
PHOTO: ERIC VON LOCKHART

BEFORE

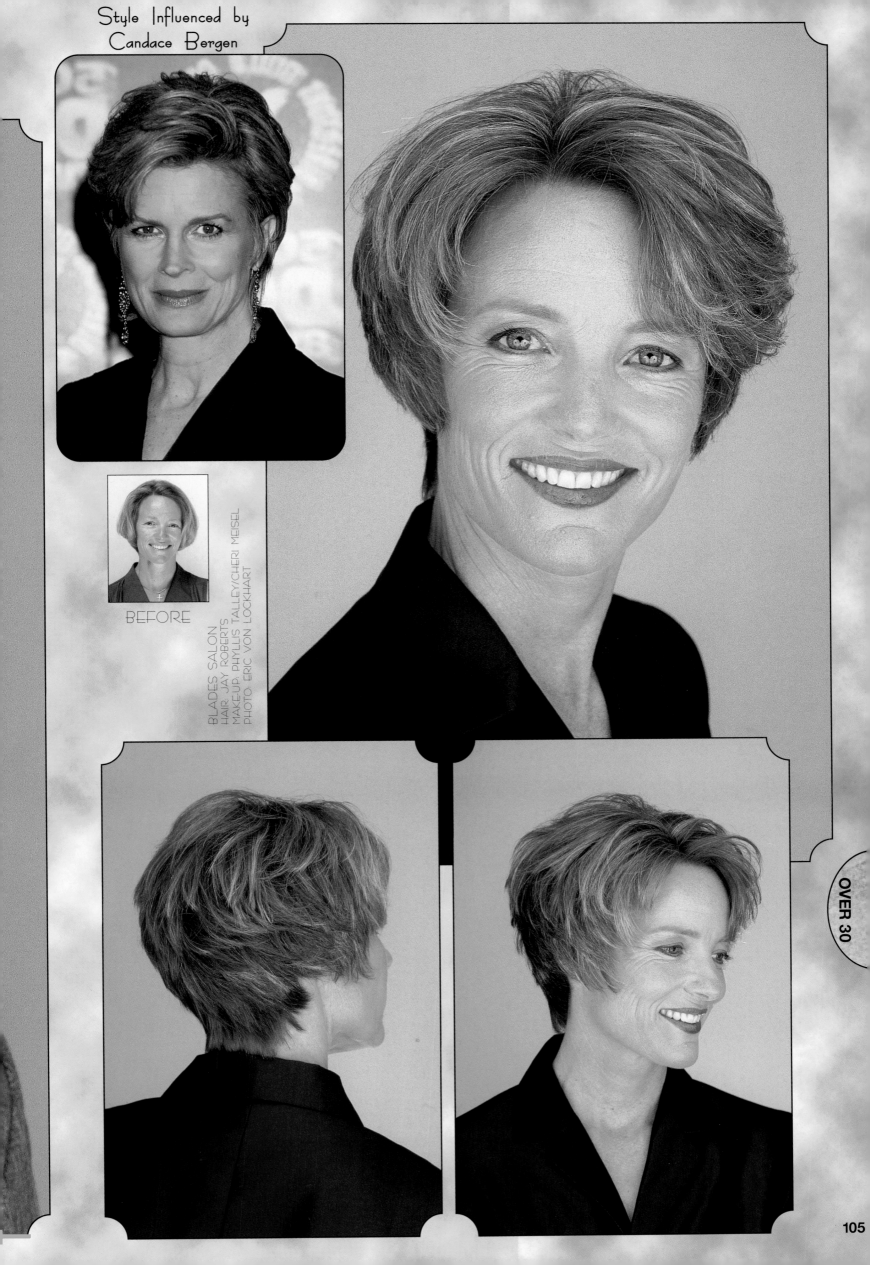

BEFORE

BLADES SALON
HAIR: JAY ROBERTS
MAKEUP: PHYLLIS TALLEY/CHERI MEISEL
PHOTO: ERIC VON LOCKHART

OVER 30

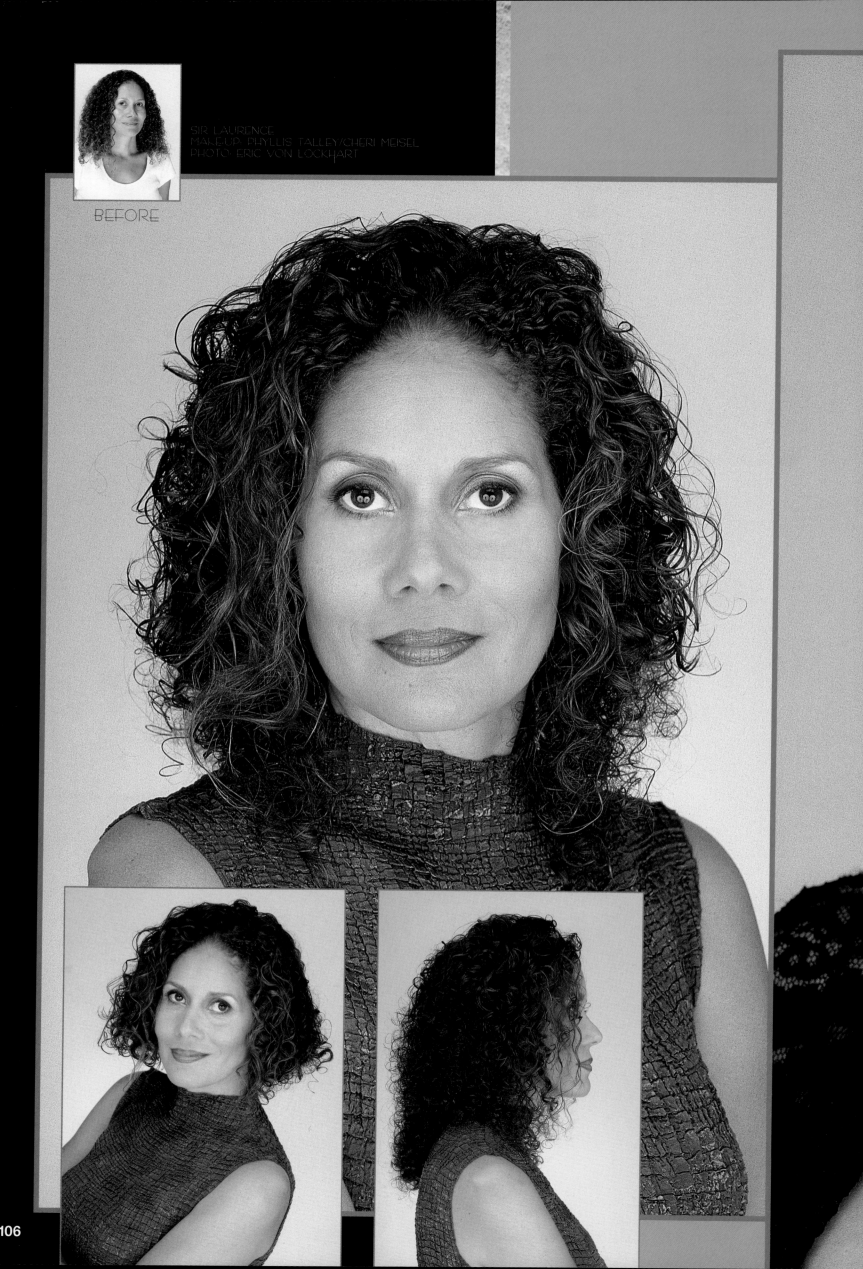

SIR LAURENCE
MAKEUP: PHYLLIS TALLEY/CHERI MEISEL
PHOTO: ERIC VON LOCKHART

BEFORE

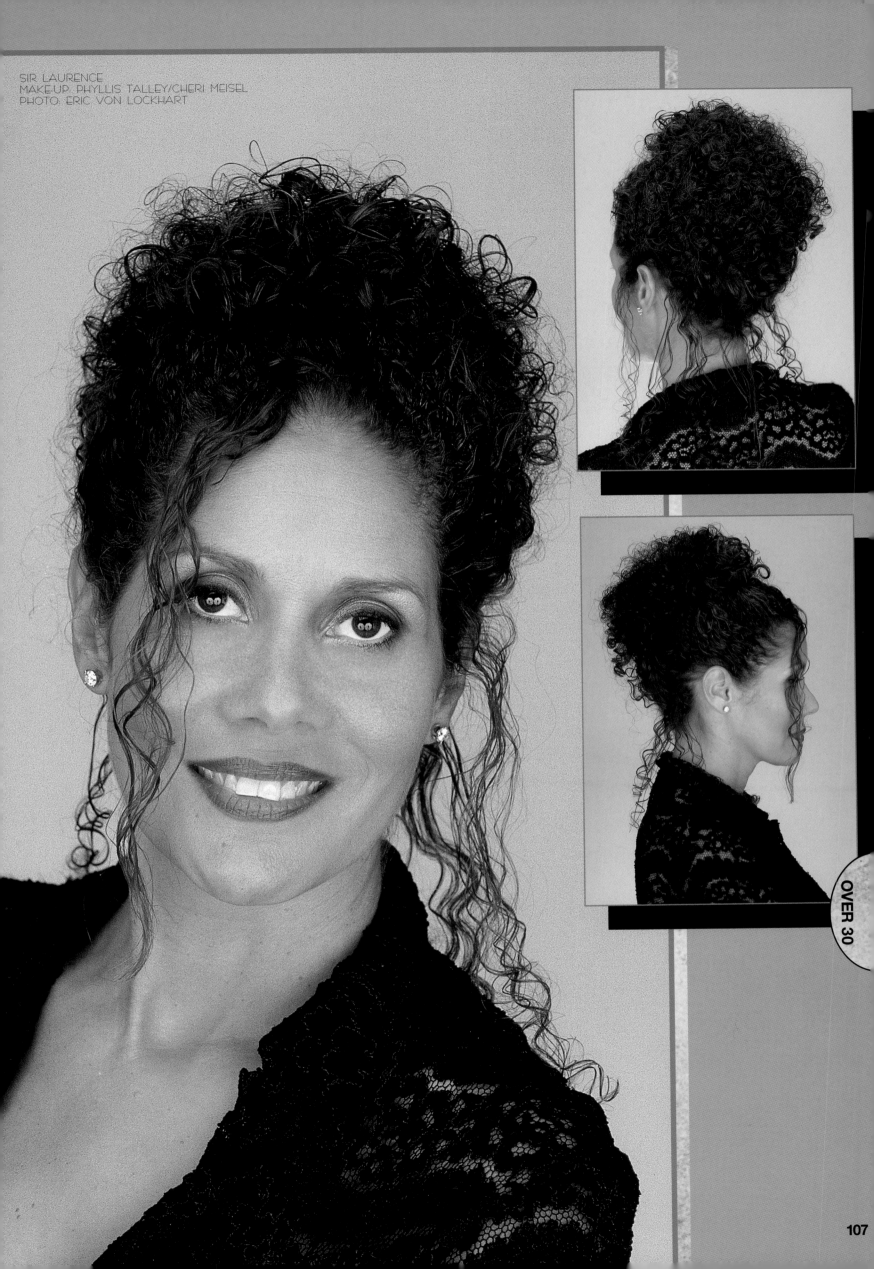

SIR LAURENCE
MAKE-UP: PHYLLIS TALLEY/CHERI MEISEL
PHOTO: ERIC VON LOCKHART

OVER 30

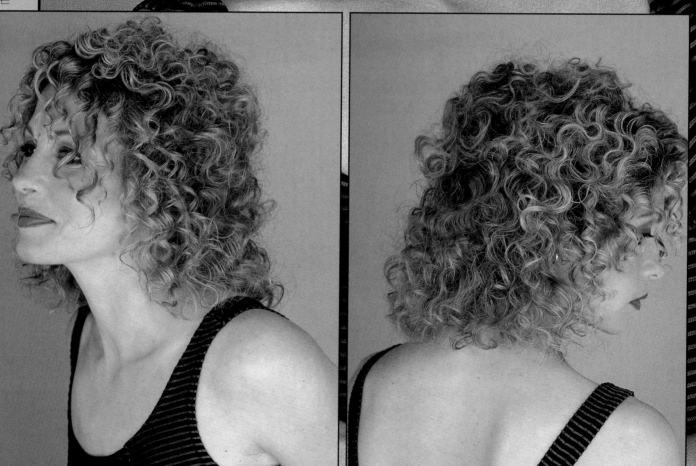

SALON MASSIMO/RENAISSANCE SALON
HAIR: MASSIMO LIGUORI/BARBARA LHOTAN
MAKEUP: PHYLLIS TALLE/CHERI MEISEL
PHOTO: ERIC VON LOCKHART

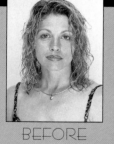

BEFORE

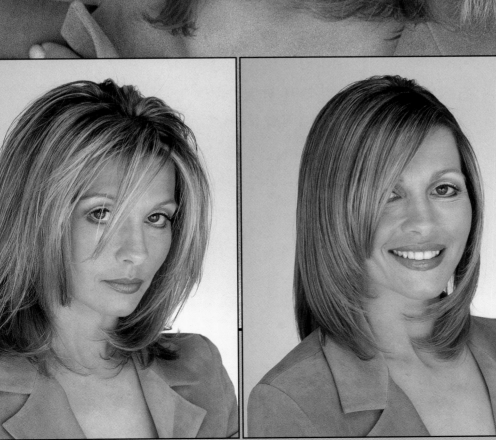

SALON MASSIMO
HAIR: MASSIMO LIGUORI
MAKE-UP: PHYLLIS TALLEY/CHERI MEISEL
PHOTO: ERIC VON LOCKHART

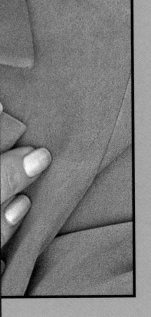

OVER 30

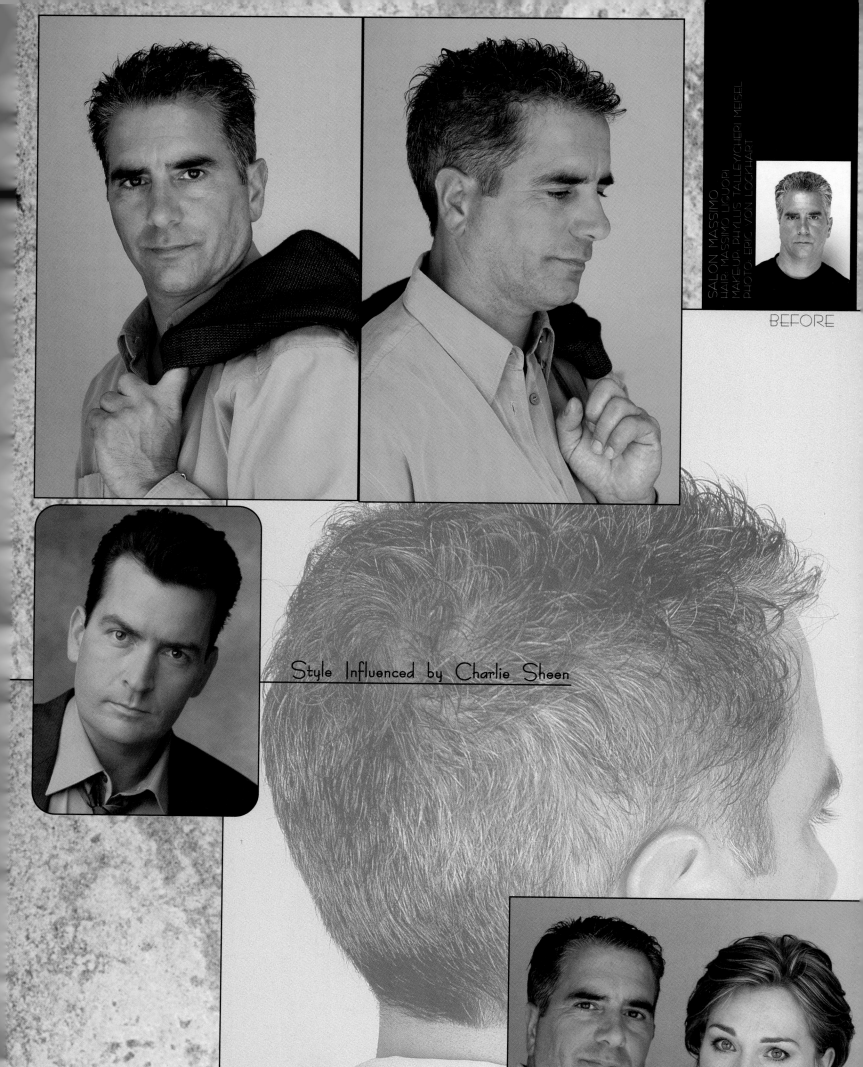

SALON MASSIMO
HAIR: MASSIMO LIGUORI
MAKEUP: PHYLLIS TALLER/CHERI MEISEL
PHOTO: ERIC VON LOCKHART

BEFORE

Style Influenced by Charlie Sheen

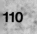

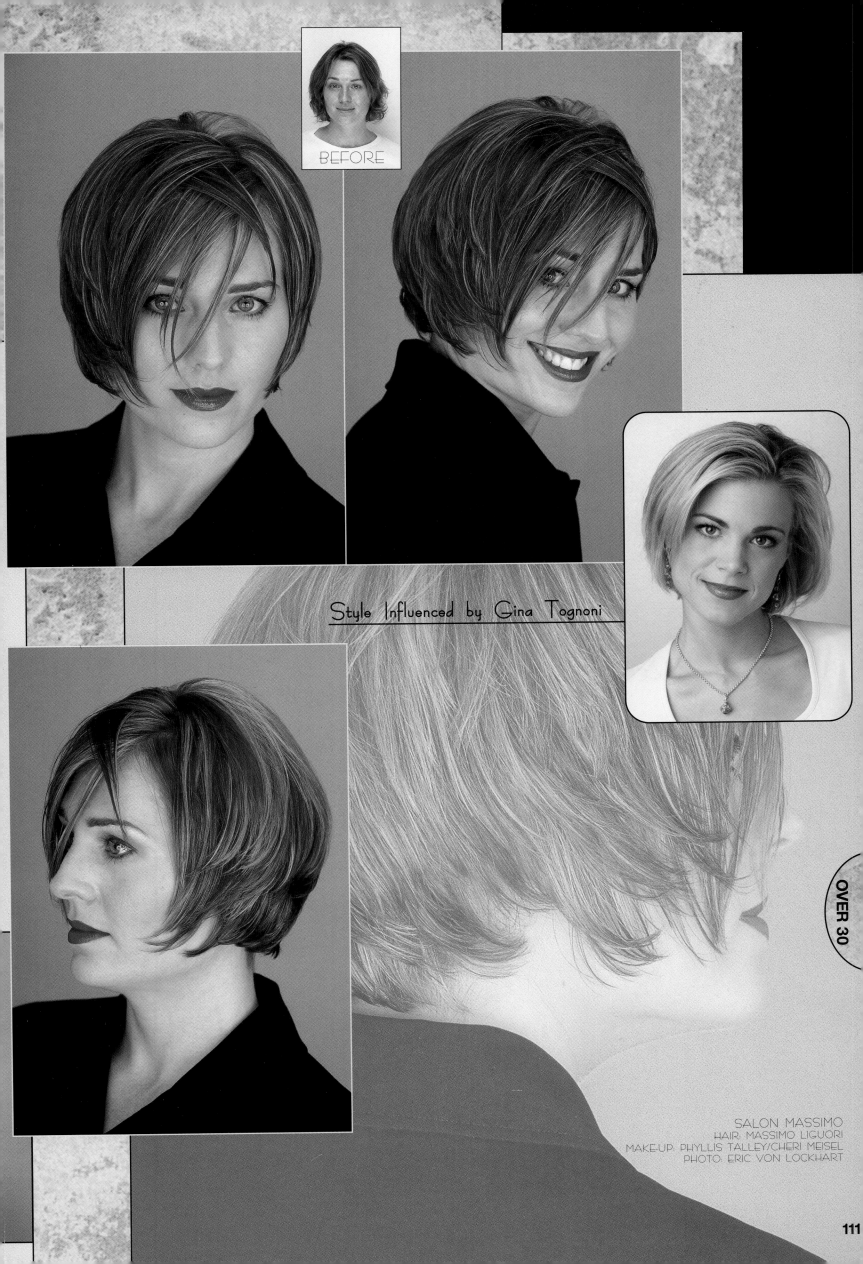

BEFORE

Style Influenced by Gina Tognoni

SALON MASSIMO
HAIR: MASSIMO LIGUORI
MAKE-UP: PHYLLIS TALLEY/CHERI MEISEL
PHOTO: ERIC VON LOCKHART

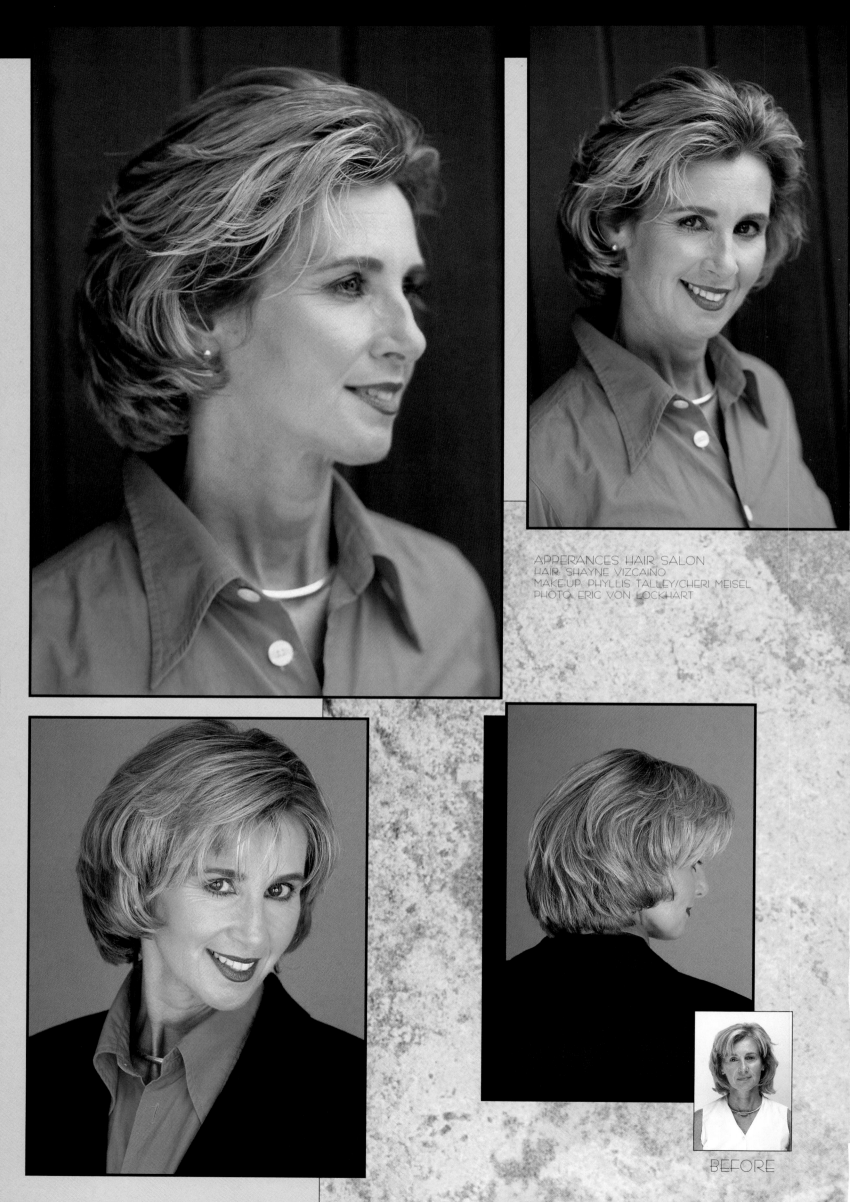

APPERANCES HAIR SALON
HAIR: SHAYNE VIZCAINO
MAKEUP: PHYLLIS TALLEY/CHERI MEISEL
PHOTO: ERIC VON LOCKHART

BEFORE

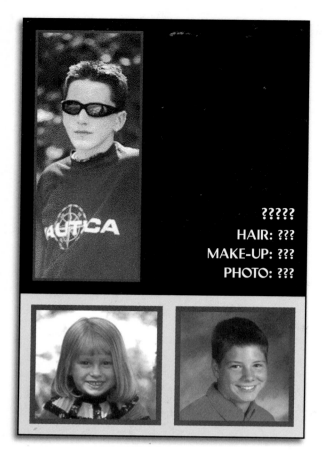

?????
HAIR: ???
MAKE-UP: ???
PHOTO: ???

What's missing from this picture?

Your Work!

INSPIRE

Bietet Ihnen in jeder Ausgabe viele Vorteile:

Immer wieder werden wir nach einem Buch gefragt, in dem alles drin ist.

Für die Beratung der Kunden braucht man im Salon normalerweise drei Bücher: Eines für die Damen, ein zweites für die Herren, und nach Möglichkeit noch eines für die Kinder.

Die INSPIRE-Frisurenbuchserie bietet eine ideale Lösung, denn in jeder Ausgabe bietet Ihnen dieses Frisurenbuch 600 Frisurenvorschläge für jeden undenwunsch.

Es gibt INSPIRE-Frisurenbücher, die zusätzlich zu den Damen-, Herren und Kinder-Frisuren noch Spezialthemen behandeln wie:

◆ Kinderfrisuren

◆ Herrenfrisuren

◆ Brautfrisuren

◆ Lady-Frisuren

◆ Teenagerfrisuren

◆ Typveränderung

Ein gut sortiertes Lager steht zu Ihrer Verfügung. Bitte fragen Sie Ihren Großhändler nach INSPIRE-Büchern.

Que manque-t-il à cette photo?

Votre Travail!

Faites publier vos photos!

Tout le monde souhaite voir ses talents et ses qualités reconnus. Quelle place pourrait être meilleure qu' INSPIRE pour vous faire connaitre?

Nous sommes intéressés de recevoir des photos de coiffures mode destinées aux clientes des salons de coiffure. Nous sommes avides de beaux modèles, de tous âges, hommes ou femmes, mais pas de travaux de haute fantaisie.

De façon à vous faire connaître, indiquez sur chaque photo: le nom du salon, le nom du coiffeur, du maquilleur, et du photographe.

S'il vous plaît n'envoyez que des dias ou négatifs couleurs de bonne qualité ou des photos noir et blanc. Joignez à chaque photo les informations précisées ci-dessus.

Vous êtes intéressé! Bravo!

Pour plus d'information sur la facon de nous transmettre vos photos, téléphonez ou écrivez à notre distributeur officiel.

Que es lo que falta en este retrato?

Tu Trabajo!

Consiga Su Trabajo Publicado!

Todo mundo tiene el deseo de que su talento y habilidades sean reconocidas.

Que mejor lugar que Inspire para recibir este reconocimiento estamos muy interesados en recibir fotografias de modas y aspectos apropiados, para la clientela de salon de belleza.

Nosotros estamos buscando modelos tanto de hombre como de mujer en cualquier edad. No queremos fotos con peinados de fantasta.

Para recibir lo anterior y darle su credito, favor de enviar fotografias muy claras, una por modelo.
Favor de enviar fotografias y/o transparencias, muy bien protegidas enviando carta, dando su permiso para la publicacion de la foto.

Esta ud interesado! Grandioso!

Para majer informacion de como enviar fotos. Formas de permiso de publicacion para posibles se iones de fotos tomadas en su area. Llamenos o escribanos para recibur guia completa.

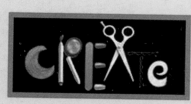